What People Are Saying About

The Nature Embedded Mind

I love the important and empowering message of psychotherapist Julie Brams' new book *The Nature Embedded Mind*. Her profound work offers us the first step in addressing the escalating, converging eco-disasters now happening on our planet. Brams urges us to wake up from the destructive delusion that humans are somehow magically separate from and superior to the rest of nature and deeply take in the reality that we are part of nature. Brams captures this simple but profound shift in thinking and inspires us to take collective, constructive healing action and to open ourselves to a profoundly joyful relationship with the rest of nature.

Linda Buzzell, LMFT, co-editor of *Healing with Nature in Mind*, researcher, author, and adjunct faculty at Pacifica Graduate Institute

In *The Nature Embedded Mind: How the Way We Think Can Heal Our Planet and Ourselves,* Brams makes a simple and inarguable case for a profound shift in thinking needed at this point in human history. Brams' recommendation of how this shift can occur, not only at the individual level but also across the entire field of Western psychology, is bold and inspirational.

Thom Hartmann, *New York Times* bestselling author of over 30 books, national and international progressive political commentator, radio personality, and talk show host

T0313497

In her book, *The Nature Embedded Mind*, Julie Brams offers a clear, inviting, and effective guidebook for coming back into direct relationship with the larger web of kinship and life that has already surrounded and sustained us. These teachings and practices are critically needed for the cultural changes ahead and support greater personal happiness and daily intimacy with body, land, and community. Highly recommended!

Daniel Foor, Ph.D., Author of *Ancestral Medicine: Rituals for Personal and Family Healing*

Julie Brams' *The Nature Embedded Mind* is a must-read for mental health clinicians in the age of the Anthropocene. As we witness the emergence of heightened climate anxiety, Brams' analysis of the intersection between eco-psychology and the practice of forest therapy stands as a beacon of hope for understanding the true medicine of the more-than-human world. Her work affirms the critical idea that repairing the relationship between humanity and the Earth is foundational to our entire experience of what we call mental health and goes beyond the idea to suggest how we can create space for the intelligence and wisdom of nature to be the source of our deepest healing.

Ben Page, author of *Healing Trees: Your Pocket Guide to Forest Bathing*, director of training for the Association of Nature and Forest Therapy, and founder of Shinrin Yoku LA and Integral Forest Bathing

The Nature Embedded Mind is an indispensable book for cultivating healing at a root level. Filled with entertaining, insightful personal stories, well-thought-out research on the intersection between environmental science and psychology, and practical methods to repair what is broken — this is a guidebook out of isolation, depression, and disconnection and towards true healing, not only of ourselves but remarkably, the entire planet. This book is a must-read for anyone seeking a future of balance, connection, and wholeness.

Marni Freedman, LMFT, program director for the San Diego Writers Festival

Julie Brams writes with great clarity and sensitivity about what it means to be a guide, and her journey to learn the art of guiding. She articulates the essential differences between guide and psychotherapist. Having trained in both practices, she is uniquely qualified to do so. She brings forward an understanding essential for all those who would be guides.

Amos Clifford, Founder CEO Association of Nature and Forest Therapy, author of *Your Guide to Forest Bathing: Experience the Healing Power of Nature*

The Nature Embedded Mind

How the Way We Think Can Heal
Our Planet and Ourselves

The Nature Embedded Mind

How the Way We Think Can Heal
Our Planet and Ourselves

Julie Brams

CHANGEMAKERS
BOOKS

London, UK
Washington, DC, USA

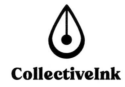

CollectiveInk

First published by Changemakers Books, 2025
Changemakers Books is an imprint of Collective Ink Ltd.,
Unit 11, Shepperton House, 89 Shepperton Road, London, N1 3DF
office@collectiveinkbooks.com
www.collectiveinkbooks.com
www.changemakers-books.com

For distributor details and how to order please visit the 'Ordering' section on our website.

Text copyright: Julie Brams 2024

ISBN: 978 1 80341 723 3
978 1 80341 791 2 (ebook)
Library of Congress Control Number: 2024931909

A CIP catalogue record for this book is available from the British Library.

Design: Lapiz Digital Services

UK: Printed and bound by CPI Group (UK) Ltd, Croydon, CR0 4YY
Printed in North America by CPI GPS partners

We operate a distinctive and ethical publishing philosophy in all areas of our business, from our global network of authors to production and worldwide distribution.

Contents

For my mom & my daughter, Marley

How to Use This Book

In brief, use this book in partnership with one or more other-than-human beings. "Other-than-human" means any of the other beings we share our world with — soil, air, water, rocks, clouds, flowers, trees, grass, squirrels, lizards, birds, bees, grasshoppers, cats, dogs, fish — the list is limitless. It also may include non-living humans, ancestors, and other spiritual beings. When you have questions, confusion, resistance or an "aha" moment, take whatever is happening in your heart out into nature and lean on another form of life to give you support and insight around the issue.

Overview

You'll get the most out of reading the chapters in order. The first few chapters outline what reEarthing means, where we've been psychologically, and where we're going, as well as defining an essential and exciting paradigm shift from seeing ourselves as separate from and dominant over nature toward perceiving ourselves as embedded in one unified collection of beings consciously interdependent upon one another. We will consider the unique role clinicians play in this paradigmatic shift and the necessary adjustment from therapist to therapist-as-guide as we expand our conscious partnership with Nature as therapist. We will explore the Association of Nature and Forest Therapy (ANFT) model of nature therapy in particular, and consider this method through my personal account, an interview with one of the original trainers/mentors of the method, as well as thoughts presented by other ANFT certified guides. We will also look at the intersection of mindfulness meditation, sensory awareness and ANFT-style nature therapy.

Each chapter includes personal anecdotes and experience, up-to-date scientific information, and reflection invitations.

The invitations are placed at breakpoints as well as at chapter endings and it's my suggestion that you stop and reflect in the moment. You may want to jot down your thoughts, and again, take whatever comes up for you in your heart and mind out into nature to receive support and insight from the more-than-human beings. In other words, take it to the woods.

FAQs

What if I'm new to this kind of information?
First and foremost, notice what resonates with you. You may already feel this perspective as true. If not, no worries. Above all, this is intended to be the start of a conversation. See what fits, ask questions, ask me, ask the trees. We're all in this together.

What if I'm not new to this kind of information?
Notice what confirms or challenges what you already think. Beginner's mind, which means approaching the information with an attitude of openness, eagerness, and lack of preconceptions, is helpful because it allows new insights, especially within areas you feel expert in. This doesn't negate your own wisdom and what you've already experienced in any way.

Additionally, this information may serve as support and validation for you in your practice and/or as a way to share these concepts with others. Whatever you find, hopefully it continues the deepening of your relationship with the rest of nature.

What if I don't live near the woods?
"Taking it to the woods" is a shorthand way of referring to all the other-than-human beings around us. If you do have woods or forest nearby with a lake, river, or stream, that's the perfect place to cultivate your relationships. If not, any outdoor setting allows us to interact with the rest of nature. We can go to a park, a beach, or our own yard. I live in an apartment and find myself

deeply connected to the palm trees, grass, insects, birds, sky, clouds, and other beings in the building's courtyard. The more-than-human world is all around us waiting to engage with us all the time.

If you feel any resistance, remember that this is most likely a sign that your mind is bumping up against the old paradigm. Take notice of it, jot it down or mark it in the book and take it to the woods. Bring whatever you're feeling (confusion, anger, fear, sadness, shame, argument, guilt) to a nature ally for help and support.

Remember, this is a centuries-old collective human bias that we're confronting. To make this shift, we all must give ourselves permission to unlearn, and relearn, as well as the permission to feel humility and recognize it as a good sign.

What Can Help

Be prepared to confront long-held pre-existing beliefs:

- about nature
- about nature therapy
- about the field of psychology
- about human evolution
- about our place in the universe
- about being an expert

Let go of your expert mind!
Again, use what is referred to in mindfulness as beginner's mind; a way of approaching without preconceptions, or prior judgment. If you have your own style of nature therapy already this may be a particular challenge. In that case, allow this to be a refresher, as well as noticing any new concepts you might like to lean into. If you don't already partner with nature, there are some simple ways to begin integrating this into your existing practice to whatever degree you feel called to do.

Keep these four core ideas close at hand:

1. Open your mind to this paradigm shift in thinking.
2. Remember this is an experiential change that requires *doing* the practice to understand it. Reading about the practice will not give you anywhere near as much appreciation as engaging in it will. Spend unstructured time in nature with whatever these ideas bring up in you.
3. Make sure you give something back to your nature allies to shift the "using nature" paradigm. Consider what you'd like to give your allies in return for what you're receiving.
4. If you're a mental health or allied professional, take your clients into the woods to support and develop their personal relationships with the other-than-humans. When you do, shift your role from therapist to guide.

Acknowledgements

My sincere gratitude for my entire publishing team at Collective Ink, Changemakers Books with special thanks to Vicky Hartley, Tim Ward, and Ben Blundell; I appreciate your belief in this message and making it possible to get it out into the world.

To my editor Marni Freedman, I honestly wouldn't have been able to do this without your unwavering support and encouragement; you are an amazing heart-mind and a dear friend. Also, to Madeleine Calvi who helped me polish my query and gave me invaluable feedback.

To the Association of Nature and Forest Therapy, M. Amos Clifford, my Southern California Forest Guide family: Ben Page, Jackie Kuang and Debra Wilbur, and Cohort 16 who helped me make my original leap into an alternate way of being with the land.

To the inspirational leaders who trailblazed this path and lit the way for me: Joanna Macy, Thom Hartmann, Linda Buzzell, Lois Arkin, John V. Davis, Theodore Roszak, Clemens G. Arvay, Thich Nhat Hanh, and so many others.

Deep love to Marley and Zack for always standing by me and encouraging me through this long journey; to Elaine who lives entirely too far away but is closer to me than anyone; to Sven for making me laugh even when I thought I couldn't; and to Mark and Arlene who were gracious enough to come on my first few nature therapy walks.

And finally immense gratitude and dedication to the many other-than-human beings, my Earth family, who support me and supported me day and night over the last seven years to deepen my understanding of this way of life. It is for them and with them that I continue to make this shift in relational consciousness.

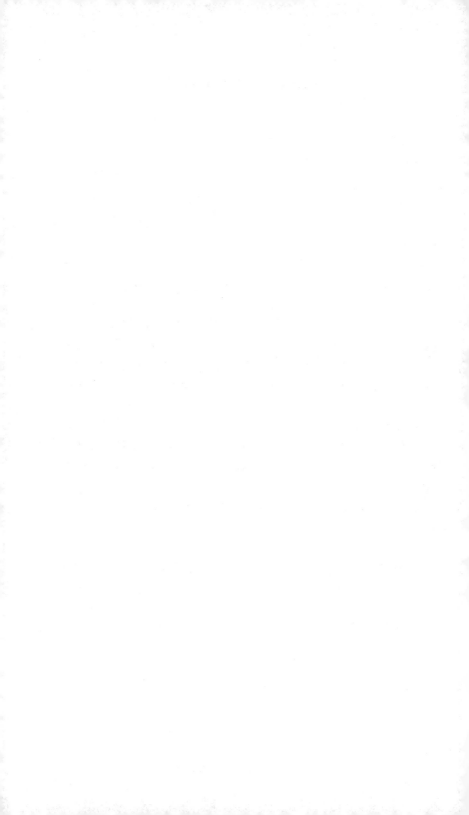

Introduction

If we are to use our tools in the service of fitting in on Earth, our basic relationship to nature — even the story we tell ourselves about who we are in the universe — has to change.

Janine Benyus, American Natural Sciences Writer, Innovation Consultant, Author

What do you notice about yourself when you lie down in the grass and gaze up at the clouds? What do you notice when you gaze into a shadowy pond long enough to discover a fish slowly moving toward you? When the sound of rustling leaves reveals a small bird nearby? What do you feel like when you sit on a boulder at the top of a mountain trail and look out at the silent trees below you? When you're brushing your dog's fur and you notice a look in his eye that you recognize as gratitude and love? What do you experience when you notice the grass in your yard is struggling in the summer heat? What do you feel when that same grass is growing lush again after you've given it more water? What happens inside you when you're walking alone in the winter woods and stop to feel the snow silently gathering on and around you? Who are you in these moments? How do you experience yourself and the world when you're in intimate connection with nature?

That you, is you in your natural consciousness, a nature embedded mind. The one you were born with.

Our knowledge about the benefits of being in nature is growing daily. Human-Nature connection plays a significant role in our health, the health of our planet, and our ability to return to a sustainable culture where humans live in balance with the rest of nature. This sustainable culture is a nature embedded way of life that stems from a nature embedded mind. This way of thinking and behaving is best exemplified by our Indigenous ancestors and our current Indigenous contemporaries. However, it's also a way of life that has no racial identity and is the natural birthright of all human beings. We are all born from Earth, and we all have the capacity to live in connection with Earth. The key to whether we do or not and to what degree we do, hinges on one simple premise in our own thinking. That premise is: I am embodied and embedded within all elements of Earth. In other words, my body is part of and connected to all the other parts of one living interdependent being named Earth.

I've written this book for many types of people. It's written for those who:

- Feel better in nature.
- Are curious about human-nature relations and what it might do for them.
- Spend most of the time indoors or online.
- Feel uncomfortable in nature.
- Want to feel better about themselves.
- Want to deepen their connections with the rest of nature.
- Are interested in ecology and practices to help the Earth.
- Are on a journey of decolonizing their mind.
- Are interested in uncovering attitudes and thoughts that may be limiting them.
- Feel deeply connected to nature and want to feel the support of others like them.

In short, it's for all of us. And it's especially written for my colleagues in mental health and allied professions since there is such a potentially unique and important role for us to play.

My hope is that this book serves as an invitation for all of us to begin an important discussion together about humans and nature, about the human mind and how it affects human behavior, about the nature of humans perhaps forgotten, and about the reclamation of our place in the natural world as a pathway to our well-being.

It's a discussion set in Rumi's grassy field "...beyond ideas of wrongdoing and rightdoing...." It is hopefully a safe space to challenge our current thinking about human-nature relations, about our personal and collective cultural assumptions, and about the role psychology plays in sustainability. Perhaps this can become a courageous space, where we consider ideas together yet come to our own conclusions, whatever they are.

I'm proposing and inviting you to join me in a significant shift in consciousness from where we are now regarding our place in nature. Yet at the same time, it's a former consciousness all our ancestors held to be true not that long ago. And it's the consciousness each of us is born with and still have. In some way, perhaps it's simply a return to our former beliefs about humans, nature, and our mutual bonds. We ourselves are nature. That is a fact. Because of that, we intrinsically have a relationship with the rest of nature whether we think we do or not. This book is simply an opportunity to look at our personal relationship with the rest of nature and assess the condition that relationship is in without judgment. You may be very pleased with what you find, and you may discover ways to be even more respectful and intimate with your more-than-human family. Or you may be startled to see how disconnected you've been from that family, so much so that you don't know how to start the conversation. That's okay too. What I hope you get from reading this book is a self-compassionate exploration of how you answer these questions with the understanding that whatever your response is, it's okay. No one knows your mind better than you. And because of that, this exploration of your own mind, your attitudes and beliefs are personal and unique to you. There are no wrong answers, only discoveries.

I'm also asking you to consider joining me in creating a shift in the field of Western psychology, not as a critique of it, or of the thousands of practitioners that use their hearts and minds each day to help people overcome mental health issues, but as an evolutionary advance in understanding consciousness. This advance is as important as the advances we've made from Freudian analysis through cognitive behaviorism, through the recent incorporation of mindfulness meditation into our therapeutic work, through neuro-therapies like EMDR Therapy and Brainspotting, and through the many somatic methods our field is still refining.

The shift I hope you will join me in making is a change in our collective premise where we regard ourselves as different from the natural world and a change in the way Western psychology currently addresses that premise. Though self-evident, the thought that we *are* nature is a thought that our minds are constantly trained away from. We're taught instead to see the human species as somehow different from the natural world and at the top of an imaginary hierarchy. Our behaviors follow that premise. Like all implicit biases, this fallacy is almost imperceptible, is self-reinstating, and needs a persistent form of intervention to make real change. Changing this assumption in our thinking is perhaps a challenge to our ego, but a crucial one at this point as we face the current crises of our time. If we succeed in making this shift, we can unlock the perceptual cages of every mind we touch and enable our species to realign itself back into a way of living that supports Earth and all its inhabitants.

We can already see this shift in thinking beginning in other professional fields (environmental sciences, biology, and business innovation), and in people in general. The global pandemic of 2020 accelerated this perceptual shift for many people as we found ourselves quarantined from each other. Questions about what was essential came to the forefront of our minds and oftentimes the answer came in the form of nature, animals, and other elements. During the pandemic, parks and beaches became literally overrun. This is the natural medicine we turned to in a time of extraordinary, never-before-seen, or experienced, stress.

You yourself may be beginning to make this shift in your consciousness. Or you may have made this shift and are now living in a consciousness where you are in respectful reciprocal relationships with the other-than-human beings around you and perceive yourself as nature. You may already be experiencing the changes that accompany that perspective. I wonder if we can embrace the potential for that same change in our mental health practices and our larger culture as well.

Another category you may notice (or be part of) is the growing number of people who can sense some kind of mental shift is needed, but not having the guidance or permission to turn to other forms of nature as equally intelligent beings, are left feeling immense fear, agitation, depression, and hopelessness about humanity and about the future of our existence. I wonder how inviting them back into their own relationship with the rest of nature might affect them.

Current scientific research shows, without a doubt, that humans are optimized in nature both physically and mentally. Studies that originated in the 1980s in Japan have now been replicated and advanced globally. Research on human health benefits associated with non-goal directed time immersed in nature shows a measurable positive effect on the immune system, cardiovascular system, stress hormones, and lifestyle diseases such as heart disease, stroke, diabetes, and cancer. Studies also find measurable psychological benefits such as stress resiliency, attention restoration, increased compassion, empathy, and creativity, and decreases in anxiety and depression. We will review the growing body of scientific research demonstrating the exact ways nature connection benefits humans, both physically and mentally. These measurable effects are encouraging and oftentimes may be the gateway for people to re-engage with nature in a meaningful way. However, it all too often stops short of the perceptual shift that we need now. Therefore, we will also look deeper into the change in consciousness we need in addition to just spending time in nature and how to reclaim our original, nature embedded consciousness easily and effortlessly.

It takes a huge act of courage to go against our collective consciousness and risk being ostracized. Science is beginning to give us the permission and courage to think differently from what we've been taught, without risking alienation from our human herd. But science is only the beginning.

With science giving us the reason why, the next step is to look at our own thinking and the actions that follow our thinking. It's only through re-engaging an intimate personal relationship with the nature around us that we can fully participate as equal members of our planetary community. Conversely to Hansel and Gretel who left breadcrumbs to find their way out of the woods, we find ourselves now stranded in our civilized, industrialized, digitized cage and needing to find the trail back into our wilderness.

The good news is that unlike Hansel and Gretel, the trail is permanently marked, doesn't disappear, cannot be destroyed, and is with you all the time. The trail back into connection with the rest of nature is your birthright. It is your own nature. Spending time in sensory connection with the rest of nature with no agenda other than to connect with the other beings, is that trail.

We will learn about an evidence-based method that allows our minds to genuinely shift the way we see ourselves in relationship with other beings. That shift in consciousness will prevent us from recreating an outdoor cage. Letting go of the idea that we are separate and different from nature is essential, though not always easy. Although it may go against our current social norms, rediscovering our personal intimate relationship with the rest of nature can be playful, fun, restful, inspiring, invigorating, pleasurable. We are hardwired for this connection yet limit ourselves by prioritizing our human-to-human connections above all others. And although we do allow ourselves to recognize interspecies connections with a small number of species we call "pets," we place an artificial limit on our ability to connect with other species. With the right guidance, nature and forest therapy provides the deep change in consciousness that can truly free us from our current thinking which has led us so far from our original way of co-existing in our planetary family.

Human history and Indigenous cultures show us examples of sustainable living; science gives us the reasons why we might want to think outside of our perceptual cage; and nature and forest therapy provides us with the way to easily shift our consciousness to a nature embedded mindset. I invite you here to take a breath and wonder with me about humans and nature. Even more to the point, about humans *as* nature: one sentient organism with many parts including, but not favoring, human beings. With that, we begin…

A Note for Clinicians and Allied Professionals:

First, I want to thank you for looking at this issue. I know how hard all of us work to serve our people and stay informed about our craft, all the while having to maintain our own balance and mental health. I've been a clinician for over 30 years now and still have a full-time, integrative private practice. I'm a mindfulness meditation practitioner and teacher and an ANFT certified forest therapy guide, but mainly I'm a fellow traveler here with you. An eternal Earth lover, a mother, a feminist, and someone who has never lost hope for the human race.

Like you, I have seen an uptick in anxiety, panic, depression, and despair in our populations, and sadly a huge spike in all the above in our children. The deep need people have seems greater than ever. It can feel daunting at times. I hope this exploration of how to lean into the intelligence of Nature as an ally in healing what ails the human mind, will refresh us as well as our worldview.

As mentioned, a primary intention for me when writing this book was to specifically call on and call-in mental health and allied professionals to join in helping a profound shift in human consciousness. As mental health professionals, we are looked to as role models and experts in what creates and sustains emotional and psychological well-being. We have the training and the skill to understand where something may be impeding a family dynamic, and we know how to listen and teach others to listen in a way that promotes bonding and harmony.

We know how and when to support our clients and we know when to step back and let healing take place. We also have permission from the people we work with to help them see things differently, to change maladaptive beliefs and to choose prosocial actions that support the holistic health of an individual, a couple, a family, or any other system.

It's already our job to help ourselves and others operate from adaptive prosocial constructs. It's already our job to find and point out maladaptive antisocial thinking. It's an exciting next step for our profession to facilitate this repair in human-nature relationship. As always, our first step is to investigate our own thinking and the actions that follow. As we learn early in our training, we can't take anyone somewhere we haven't been ourselves. So, grab your courage, and your curiosity. It's time to expand our thinking again. This time with regards to our relationship with nature, the other-than-human beings with whom we share and co-create our world. Then we can begin helping our clients' relationships with nature. It's already our job to help heal relationships. It's simply a matter of expanding our sense of family to include the other-than-human beings, the rest of nature.

I invite you to come along on this journey, to examine how we see ourselves in relationship to the rest of nature. I invite you to learn about and explore the Association of Nature and Forest Therapy (ANFT) style of nature therapy in particular, because of its standardized methodology. I promise you that this exploration will be fun and relaxing all the while changing how you see yourself as a member of Earth. Though this is not a training manual, notice if what you discover here prompts you to consider how your own practice of or certification in ANFT-style forest therapy may shift or enhance your beliefs about mental health and your practice.

Finally, I invite those of you in healing professions to join me in helping your clients reconsider their beliefs about themselves and nature and experience the changes that occur when they are guided by you to repair and reconnect this most precious and crucial relationship.

There has been no greater time in history than now to confront the faulty premise that humans are something other than and outside of the rest of nature. It's my hope that this book will allow us to explore and wonder about this premise, how it may operate in our perception of ourselves and nature, and perhaps recognize what behaviors might change as our perceptions expand. And lastly, give us an effortless desire to help our clients confront it in themselves as well. In this way, we can heal. And in our healing, we have a chance and opportunity to return to a sustainable way of living *in* our planet, not on it.

1

My Journey: Stepping Down off the Pedestal and reEarthing Myself

You only have to let the soft animal of your body love what it loves.

Mary Oliver, American poet

My journey of living a nature embedded life and bringing it into my clinical work has been, and still is, a constant practice of thinking, rethinking, and challenging my beliefs. Oftentimes it's embarrassing to uncover yet another hidden bias or habit I have that either keeps me thinking and acting like I'm separate from the rest of nature, or that I'm superior to another being, especially the ones I don't like, mosquitos for example. I've found this path to be repeatedly humbling yet also funny. As a child I really disliked teasing; I didn't get it. But as an adult, I see the value of teasing in that it can break an overly self-serious attitude. Some of the observations I share may come from that sense of humor. I hope you can enjoy it in the spirit that it's intended. The idea of stepping down off the pedestal is one of those images for me. It pokes fun at myself and our species for placing humans above the rest of nature. The emperors with our beautiful new clothes.

However, on a deeper level, if you let it sink in, it also speaks to the artificial pressure we have put on ourselves to have all the answers and the relief we can enjoy knowing we aren't the only intelligent beings on the planet to help solve our problems. If you've ever been put on a pedestal, you know how limiting and rigid an experience that is. Stepping down off the pedestal as a species means we can relax into a shared experience where all the others are also allowed to contribute. Nature-inspired innovation in business is already firmly in place as sustainable living has become a global human intention. Biomimicry is just one example of how the rest of nature has a lot to offer us in terms of solutions to our complex human problems. And yet, as a species, we still tend to think in a way that works against ourselves. This is where I believe a movement to reEarth our thinking, our psychology, is as promising as it is essential.

Why use the word reEarthing and what does it mean? reEarthing is a way of thinking about ourselves in relationship with nature. reEarthing shifts our self-perception so that we acknowledge ourselves as part of nature, part of the whole, not better than nor worse than any other part.

When we reEarth ourselves we begin to experience that we are in partnership with all beings, and that we have a role in the natural world equal to but not greater than our Earthmates, that we *are* Earth. I chose to use lowercase letters for "re" because I want to highlight that, whether we *think* we are Earth or not, we are. There's no way for us not to be Earth. It's simply whether we make that reality conscious or not and to what degree.

Everyone already has a "reEarthed" self. For instance, when we feel the urge to water drooping plants, or enjoy our dog greeting us at the door, or inhale oxygen and exhale carbon dioxide, we are engaging from our reEarthed self. By contrast, when we take a walk down the block to grab a coffee while talking on the phone and cut across a lawn to save time, we are in our nature-disconnected self. Our mind has reverted to thinking that we are separate from the other beings and therefore our actions don't include them or our relationship with them. Grass, in this case, becomes a surface I am walking on. Even in our reEarthed self we may cut across the grass, but the experience will be different when we keep our relationship with the grass in mind. What that difference is will be unique to you and will depend on the relationship you've cultivated with the grass. Whether you like the experience more or less than your nature-disconnected self is up to you to discover as well.

One of the first considerations in reEarthing is how we talk about ourselves and the natural world. For example, the sentence I just used is nature-disconnected. It separates "us" from "the natural world." A nature embedded, or reEarthed, sentence would be: One of the first considerations in reEarthing is how we talk about ourselves *and the rest of nature*. This sentence acknowledges and includes us as one of the many forms of nature and recognizes our relationship with the other forms. Nature-disconnected language reinforces the artificial split. It becomes starkly apparent in the language we use daily. Seemingly benign phrases like "I'm going out into nature this weekend," "I'd love to own land," "I'm not really a nature person," "being in nature is good for your health," reveal the core human-nature separated premise that we build the rest of our beliefs and behaviors on. Paying attention to and changing the language we use is an important beginning in how we can align our thinking with a nature embedded premise. The use of nature embedded language throughout this book might sound odd, uncomfortable, or confusing at first. If it does, that's simply an opportunity to reflect on the dissonance the language is causing with a pre-existing nature-separated thought. Dissonance and discomfort can be useful allies to us when it comes to making deep changes. It can also feel difficult and discouraging at times.

Two other terms I will use throughout the book are "more-than-human beings" and "other-than-human beings." These terms simply refer to any of the millions of other beings we share every moment of our lives with — animals, insects, microbes, plants, minerals, water, air, fire to name broad categories — and allow us to decenter human beings as we reEarth our thinking and nature embed our minds.

If you decide you'd like to explore this mindset, be gentle with yourself. We've been taught to think in a nature-separated way for a very long time. It structures our world and directs what we believe about human beings, our place in relationship with other-than-humans and our human potential itself.

One simple example of this is our storytelling in literature, film, and television. Man versus Nature is often the theme pitting humanity against other beings or going to incredible lengths to survive the wilderness. Although the wilderness does require respect and certain skills, the idea that we are at war with our environment and must conquer nature is a human-created concept. This conflict-driven relationship is not limited to entertainment. It's a framework that our humanity works within all the time, consciously, unconsciously and to greater or lesser degrees. It shapes, and limits, what we believe to be true about our species.

Because of that, it's important to consider looking at and perhaps challenging our collective conceptions about human nature. Arguments about human nature, our fundamental dispositions, ways of thinking, feeling, and behaving have been debated for centuries.

Historically, in Western psychology theories about human behavior and development, mental health or mental illness centered around the question of what is intrinsic in a person and what is learned through childrearing practices and cultural experiences. Eventually, Western psychology settled on an explanation acknowledging that a combination of both results in a person's thoughts and behaviors, and whether they are considered functional and adaptive or dysfunctional and maladaptive. For the purposes of our exploration, I'd like to consider all hypotheses about human nature and the common ways we have of thinking about the human species rather than getting into a philosophical debate about which perspective is correct. I'd like us to wonder together about all our assumptions about human nature, because mainly we're evaluating behavior that's occurring post-civilization. We're observing behavior that results from a nature-separated mindset.

The merging of theological and philosophical arguments brought forth ideas of inherent goodness with two categories of belief: humans are innately "basically good" or humans are innately "basically sinful, self-centered and corrupt." Most people still tend to talk about human nature in this way especially when confronted by antisocial behaviors, from lying and stealing to horrific abuse and violence. It's hard to make sense of the ways we mistreat each other, the way we mistreat other species, and the way we mistreat our environment.

Although I tend to fall in the former group, that people are innately good, I have had countless experiences of people pointing out the horrific things people do as evidence to the contrary. It certainly can feel like a losing battle. Oftentimes we tell each other a lot of stories about human nature when we see behavior that is cruel. Stories about aggression, violence, destruction, jealousy, oppression, greed, and a host of other antisocial qualities are explained as inevitable because, "That's how it's always been. It's human nature." Even a person who believes in innate goodness may want to throw in the towel on the human race.

The antisocial qualities and behaviors humanity seems unable to stop would suggest it's something about our nature. But what I'd like us to wonder about is, are these qualities truly natural to us? Or are they the result of living in a perceptual paradigm and social structure that goes against our nature? We have no doubt that animals living in captivity behave differently than in their natural environment, or as we say, "in the wild." For example, many chimpanzees in captivity show a variety of serious behavioral abnormalities, some of which have been considered as possible signs of compromised mental health. These are behaviors that don't occur in chimps living in their natural environment. And studies show that Beluga whales in captivity show aggressive behavior as their only means of expressing their distress and suffering in situations they cannot escape. In the case of Beluga whales, people have misattributed the behavior to "playfulness," but marine biologists have no doubts that the Belugas are showing behaviors that do not occur in the wild and are symptomatic of distress.

Is it possible that humans are in this same predicament? In the case of our own species, not only do we have trouble recognizing how captivity has changed human behavior, but we can't even perceive that we are captive. And we, like in the case of Belugas, may have some gross misinterpretations of what is normal, expected, and acceptable. We've been living in captivity for generations upon generations. For so long, in fact, we don't remember what non-captivity is like. When we imagine the alternative to the life we've grown accustomed to, we default to fictional and mythological descriptions that are usually negative or frightening to us. Something like living in a cave somewhere vulnerable to the elements and wild animals. If we tell ourselves that a nature embedded lifestyle is scary, threatening, and difficult to survive, we won't even allow ourselves the chance to imagine what it might actually be like, much less engage in ways that would create such a lifestyle. Which, by the way, keeps us in captivity.

The captivity that I'm referring to is simply the perceptual cage we call civilization. Civilization describes itself as distinctly different from what in the past was insultingly referred to as "savage" or "wild" cultures that were being colonized. Truthfully, pre-colonized Indigenous cultures were and are a way of life humans developed by living in intimate connection and respectful harmony with the rest of nature. In fact, nature embedded cultures have survived sustainably for thousands of years.

Civilization distinguishes itself by fundamentally denying our human-nature connection. Its denial begins at the personal level and extends to the larger societal level. The civilization that we're a part of right this minute is functioning on that premise and we, as part of that structure, are functioning in that denial along with it. Right this minute you and I are functioning in a society that denies our deepest connection with Earth. We may have an intellectual understanding that we are part of Earth, just as the soil is. Yet we perceive ourselves as separate from soil, maybe even better or more important than soil. Certainly, more intelligent, right? We don't usually think about the fact that our bodies include some of the same elements as soil, or that the soil in part transforms into the fruits and vegetables we eat. To belong and function in this society, we suspend those thoughts and operate with the contradictory premise that we are different from the rest of nature and therefore separate from it.

When we maintain this distorted perceptual barrier that we are different from, superior to, or sometimes inferior to the rest of nature, and these same beliefs have created a lifestyle where we rarely have access to our original habitat, how can we possibly claim to know what is natural in humans? It's quite possible that what we know of ourselves now is solely how we behave within the limits of a social structure founded on that false premise. Little by little we have left behind Nature itself and what we may have known as our natural way of being.

When we engage in a practice to restore our original sense of "Self-as-Earth," recognizing that humans and nature are the same thing, we can repair our fundamental human-nature connection, that intrinsic bond, and regain a sense of how we belong in and to nature. Then we can rediscover how we behave naturally, meaning in alignment with our true untamed human nature, as well as in alignment with the rest of nature with which we co-create and co-inhabit our planet.

My personal reEarthing process began one afternoon in 2005 while reading Thom Hartmann's book, *The Last Hours of Ancient*

Sunlight. I embraced his thoughts on the unsustainability of living in our modern fossil fuel-based, consumption-oriented culture in contrast to the Indigenous cultures of our ancestors who lived sustainably for tens of thousands of years. This truth challenged what I had been taught, that our technological advances from the cotton gin to the internet made us better as a society and had overpowered, colonized, or otherwise "wiped out" nature-based cultures.

However, that's not true. We don't have to travel back in time to find examples of nature embedded people. Nor have these people been wiped out. There are an estimated 476 million Indigenous people in the world. Seven million live just in the United States. The United American Indians of New England proudly remind all of us, "We Are Not Vanishing. We Are Not Conquered. We Are Strong As Ever." There are also thought to be around 100 uncontacted tribes living in hard-to-reach areas around the world. These people, experts in living in the forests, are well aware of the "outside world," yet choose to stay independent from civilization, preferring their way of life deep in the forest.

There are tribal people choosing voluntary isolation in the rainforests of Brazil. These people are nomadic and live by fishing and hunting. They keep themselves separate from loggers and others that pose modern threats. Dwellings can be built in a matter of hours and provide shelter for the tribe for as long as needed and then are left behind as they move deeper into the forest when outsiders threaten to make contact. Other uncontacted tribes are protected by the government and no contact is made unless there is some danger to the tribes. These uncontacted people live in harmony with the rest of nature as well as with neighboring tribes, with whom they may or may not have friendly relations.

There are also Indigenous cultures that have escaped colonization and therefore still carry the wisdom of their ancestors and a lifestyle that is in harmony with the rest of nature. One example is the Aboriginals in the Australian outback. Experts in living in areas that colonizers couldn't survive in, they have been able to maintain themselves and their way of life. And, despite colonization, other Indigenous cultures in the Americas and Africa have maintained the wisdom of their (our) ancestors and their wisdom traditions.

You may be wondering if the goal of repairing our human-nature relationship means going back to an ancient way of life and leaving our modern technology behind. The simple answer is no. However, understanding the results of separating ourselves from the rest of nature is important for our species and ultimately for creating a new way of sustainable living. Finding a way of reintegrating ourselves back into alignment with the rest of nature is perhaps the process of defining a new culture, a third way, which serves us all, human and more-than-human alike. The most significant changes will be in our mind, perceptual and internal. The external result, meaning how that culture will behave, will unfold from there. Each of us will be part of what that new way looks like.

Back to that sunny afternoon in 2005 and Thom Hartmann's *The Last Hours of Ancient Sunlight*. Hartmann distinguishes two cultures that can begin to orient our inner guidance system, Older Culture and Younger Culture. Hartmann (2004) states, "Older Culture tells a story where all things have value and a sacred right to live on this planet while Younger Culture is based on the story that humans are the 'master species' and should be served by everything else."

As I contemplated those two premises that day, I recognized where my truth existed. The idea that humans are, or should be, the master species never rang true for me, but until then I had never connected it to the concept of environmental sustainability. Somewhere deep inside me, a knowing stirred. It was as if a small singular voice inside me since childhood was suddenly given the reason for its existence and an amplifier: Everything on Earth is valuable and has a sacred right to life. Interconnectedness is how we thrive. Our humility will determine our survival. Our collective story will determine our fate.

Our collective story about our place in nature, our thinking, is the key to changing not only how we experience life here, but whether we will survive as a species.

Reflection Invitation

I invite you to notice what comes up in you when you think of a new paradigm that decenters humans and recognizes and respects the interconnection of all beings as equally critical to a healthy whole. If this is challenging, what do you notice is problematic? Do you believe that humans are the "master species" and should be served by everything else? Why or why not?

As a child, I had an affinity, respect, and preference for Indigenous culture over the dominant culture within which I was raised. I believed that modern social norms were experimental ideas at best and harmful at worst. So much of what I saw in human behavior made no sense to me. I tried to see my world through Indigenous eyes if possible or through animal eyes to expand my understanding of what was healthy. I continue to look to Indigenous tradition as much as possible and to the other-than-human world for guidance. One example that may raise some eyebrows was motherhood. In considering how to care for my baby, I looked to primate motherhood to help me. Recognizing that my human culture had experimented with and recommended infant parenting techniques like letting an infant "cry itself to sleep" seemed completely shocking to me. Turning to other-than-human guidance, I chose feeding on demand, carrying my baby as much as possible, and sleeping with her as other primates (and, I imagined, most mammals) would do in order to keep their offspring safe from predators. Although there is still a pressured debate about whether to sleep with your babies, many tribal people co-sleep with family members, and all people, tribal or not, practiced co-sleeping until the thirteenth century. Turning to the more-than-human world for advice, I opted for an Older Culture way with confidence. Twenty-eight years later, I can attest that this style created a healthy, independent woman.

A nature-informed way of life has always felt more comfortable, and less stressful. Perhaps you also share that experience, and if not, that's all right. Growing up, my schools taught me some things about Indigenous ways from a positive perspective. However, I was also taught to believe that those ways were destroyed, lost, or forgotten. My history classes right through college described Indigenous life as ideal, yet destined to be massacred, overthrown, or contaminated by "progress." After all, what human could possibly resist what modern life has to offer, especially once they've been taught that things go better with Coke?

At the time of writing this, these cultural myths are being challenged with new vigor. As Black, Indigenous and People of Color are demanding real equity, schools are beginning to change their curriculum to reflect the truth about diverse cultures and the truth about White privileged culture. Unmasking and challenging White supremacy and colonization and engaging in the processes of decolonization, diversity, equity, and inclusion, these groups of people are making further headway in changing mainstream consciousness.

In my upbringing, however, I bought into the myth that the dominant culture would somehow always destroy Indigenous wisdom, whether intentionally or unintentionally, much to my frustration and despair. I also bought into the myth that somehow Indigenous ways were foreign, reserved for certain races, "not White" and therefore, would have to be learned like a foreign language or forbidden for me. Those two myths prove false as well. As I contemplated how to rediscover an Older Culture way of thinking about our place in the rest of nature, it dawned on me that the older way is the natural way, for all of us. The older way is embedded in our DNA, embedded in our bodies, regardless of race or culture. It's our birthright and is what makes us human. It can't be taken away from us, destroyed, or erased. The only thing standing in our way, is our way of thinking. And thinking, as we know, can be changed. If we recognize this critical need to shift the human psyche back into a paradigm that decenters the human species and embrace it again as our collective premise, we should be able to effortlessly take actions that truly respect and support all life. In that moment, a fire was lit in me that I could not douse, nor, I might add, did I have any inclination to want to.

As mental health professionals, we have a clear understanding that humans are storytellers. We make meaning about ourselves, our relationships and our world through the narratives, the thoughts, beliefs, and ideas we teach each other. Our thoughts shape our world. Our thoughts inform our actions and our choices. And to change our actions, our behavior, we need to change our thinking. Thom Hartmann highlights these points:

Ideas preceded every revolution, every war, every transformation, and every invention. So, the good news is that if we redefine our cultural norms, retell the stories that make up the reality we follow, then humanity's behaviors will change to conform to the new stories.

Younger cultures are still an experiment, and every time one has been attempted (Sumer, Rome, Greece), however great its grandeur, it has self-destructed, while tribes survive thousands of years.

Older cultures are most often cooperators, not dominators.

There are human cultures who do not engage in the destruction of the world. They demonstrate that destruction and domination are not an inevitable part of human nature.

About 7000 years ago, the anthropological record shows that not one culture believed itself to be separate from and superior to nature ... we enjoyed cradle-to-grave security. The tribe took care of itself, we cared for one another. If anybody had food, everybody had food; if anybody had a diseased child or an infirm parent, everybody had a diseased child or an infirm parent.

The measure of wealth in such societies was security. Mediums of exchange like money were unnecessary; the idea of hoarding food or other things was unthinkable because everybody was responsible for everybody.

What we must remember is the older culture view: We are part of the world, and it is our destiny to cooperate with the rest of creation. (*The Last Hours of Ancient Sunlight*, p.177.)

What struck my heart as I read those words was the simple premise that we need to tell a different story. An older story. A story that sustains us.

Reflection Invitation

"It is our destiny to cooperate with the rest of creation."

I invite you to consider what that idea brings up for you. Can you imagine what it means for humans to cooperate with the rest of creation? How do you see yourself in terms of cooperating with the rest of creation? Do you see any examples of man against nature stories in your personal storytelling or in books and movies? What do you notice in the language you hear and use regarding nature?

2

Possibilities: Reclaiming Our Natural Mind

If the world is to be healed through human efforts, I am convinced it will be by ordinary people, people whose love for this life is even greater than their fear.
Joanna Macy, American activist, author, scholar

We can see our natural world straining to balance-correct under human-made problems stemming from this foundational split we've made between ourselves and the rest of nature. We can also feel the strain in our own bodies in excessive anxiety, panic, depression, illness, and fatigue since no matter what we think, our bodies remain connected to Earth, and our bodies experience the same imbalances the rest of the planet does. The good news is that with intentional practice the divide in our psyche can be mended. Our deep recognition, and our felt sense of the truth that we are ourselves nature, will bring us back to our natural way of living indivisibly.

However, the healing we need is more than just telling a different story simply by re-wording it. It's an experiential healing. A practice. Focusing on thinking alone as a means to profound change is limited. Deep and lasting change comes through our whole bodies in connection with our thoughts. The process of change that can heal this psychic tear necessitates an actual shift in consciousness through the felt sense of interconnection to the rest of nature. It was then that I set out to find the how. In other words, an evidence-based, standardized method of mending our relationship with the other-than-humans and cultivating our self-perception as Nature.

I remember sitting in my upstairs bedroom in Porter Ranch, California thinking, "There must be a way for me to use my skillset as a mental health professional to help people make a mental shift to sustainability." My daughter, Marley, 9 years old at the time, was playing lawn surfing with her best friend, Nikki. They would take an old cardboard box and slide down the small grassy hill just below my window. It was the perfect situation where they felt all the freedom and independence of playing alone outside, while I could keep my eyes and ears on them from above. As I watched these two beautiful girls play, I allowed myself to imagine the probability that their future held what I envisioned as an apocalyptic fight for the world's remaining oil replete with wars, famine, genocide, and a kind of global looting as the modernized human culture toppled over. That idea was enough to keep me searching the literature as well as my own heart and mind for another way for our human story to play itself out.

It was with that dedication that I began my foray into the sub-field of Ecopsychology, a term coined by scholar Theodore Roszak, in 1992; yet still so emergent that it is constantly underlined for auto spell-check. If you are familiar with Roszak and the field of Ecopsychology feel free to skim or skip this chapter or come along for a refresher.

Published in 1995, Roszak's compilation of essays *Ecopsychology: Restoring the Earth, Healing the Mind*, brought together several voices on the topic of the human-nature relationship and its primary role in mental health and environmentalism. These ideas set a foundation for considering the role that nature plays in human health and established some clear principles. We will explore these concepts in the next chapter. In brief, Ecopsychology recognizes that human wellness is interdependent with nature. In other words, we cannot truly be well if our environment isn't well. Remember we are one and the same. If we go that one step further in our consciousness and recognize we *are* our environment, not separate from it, of course we can't.

Reflection Invitation

I invite you to consider what the idea of a Human-Nature relationship means to you both personally and/or professionally if you are a clinician. Have you thought about the role this relationship plays in your mental health?

Roszak's work led me to other people's writings, and although I found plenty of philosophical information, it was harder to find anything that really outlined a standardized method of bringing these concepts into the therapy room. Most experts in Ecotherapy, I found, were mavericks, creating ways of bringing people and nature together. Ecotherapy was seen as a frontier and experimentation was the course of action, but I didn't feel comfortable as a trailblazer. Some of you may be those mavericks and, if so, I tip my hat to you. I admire your courage and creativity and am very interested in what you discovered.

For my own comfort level, I wanted to know that what I was doing was something already verified, researched, and as guaranteed as possible to create the cognitive shift I believed was necessary. I found myself resonating completely with the ideas but stumped about how to even bring the concepts up with colleagues, clients, or anyone for that matter, much less help them engage in a therapeutic method that would provide actual healing.

I came to understand two basic social organizations humans use: Tribes and City-states. Tribes are cooperative, independent, egalitarian, use renewable resources, have a unique sense of identity and a respect for other tribes' identity; in other words, they value diversity.

City-states use domination, hierarchy, conquest, absorption or assimilation of conquered peoples, and warfare. In our world, City-states exist, and may be here to stay. However, we can build communities that work with tribal values. We can form, and are forming, new "tribes" in the form of intentional communities where people care for each other and live sustainably. We can even see these values entering the workforce with organizational structures that are replacing the old corporate model. What appealed to me most about this way of thinking is that it moves us forward organically. It's exciting to imagine what our current structure may become when we reinstate tribal values. I started exploring what I could find around the concept of modern tribes and villages.

According to anthropologist Robin Dunbar, groups of people organize and maintain themselves cohesively if the number of people is around 150 or less (Dunbar's number). My understanding is that once the number of people in the group grows past that, the stability of the system begins to break down as the members become less connected emotionally and morally to one another. In my mind, the implications that followed were that larger groups begin to use more restrictive rules, laws, and norms to attempt to maintain stability and cohesion. I was fascinated by this idea of a human nature where we behaved pro-socially without much intervention, simply because we felt for each other. And again, if we also include the more-than-human beings in our tribe, our behavior would be quite different from what it is now. I wondered who might be practicing this kind of intentional community living and discovered two places that drew my attention: Damanhur in Italy and a place called the Los Angeles Eco-Village. My heart was set on Italy, but sadly my pocketbook wasn't.

The next weekend I took the girls out and we went on a tour of the Los Angeles Eco-Village nestled in the north end of the Wilshire Center/Koreatown area of Los Angeles, consisting of two blocks of Bimini and White House Place. This intentional community holds seven core values:

- Celebrate and include joy in all our endeavors.
- Take responsibility for each other and the planet through local, environmental and social action.
- Learn from Nature and live ecologically.
- Build a dynamic community through diversity and cooperation.
- Inspire compassionate, nurturing, respectful relationships.
- Create balanced opportunities for individual participation and collective stewardship.
- Engage our neighbors and broader communities in mutual dialogue to learn, teach and act.

I was encouraged. Here was a functioning village of sorts where its members operated cooperatively for a common good and demonstrated sustainable urban living. I was surprised to find that the village consisted of around 40 people who resided in two neighboring apartment buildings. We arrived at the main building to meet the founder, Lois Arkin, who was also our tour guide. The building was a charming, multi-family structure whose residents were re-imagining into a village. The village was achieved through shared physical space and intentionality. For example, the ground floor provided a communal living room, food co-op, and bike repair shop that residents passed through on the way to their own apartments. I was told that this design gave plenty of opportunity for residents to feel connected to each other and to spend time together. The bike shop provided people with a way of transportation as well as income. The land in the courtyard provided gardens for anyone interested in growing. Several fruit and nut trees were intentionally planted to provide food. A spacious chicken coup also allowed residents to share in the eggs and the care of the birds. Many of the villagers contributed to the community through small sustainable businesses. Others contributed to the village's Time Bank, a system that values everyone's time equally (one hour equals one credit) and allows exchange of time credits for other goods and services. Decision-making about the buildings, and the land around them, was made communally, each member having an equal voice about what should or shouldn't be done. It was fascinating and functioning. I recently had the pleasure of speaking with Lois again and learned that the village, now in its thirtieth year, has expanded to include projects ranging from soil healing on a parcel of land that was polluted by a former auto shop, to developing a fully off-grid tiny home, to providing the community and surrounding areas with mobile karaoke experiences and other educational and play opportunities. It is still awe-inspiring to see what this intentional community is modeling in terms of sustainability, self-sufficiency, ecological sensitivity, and cooperation among people of all ages and all walks of life.

Reflection Invitation

I invite you to wander out into the rest of nature and notice what comes up when you imagine the possibility of a healed culture. Do you notice any resistance to the possibility? Do you notice any part of you that starts to create a scenario where you and the people around you return to a way of thinking about life where all beings are respected and included in the actions taken?

Toward the end of our tour, Lois asked me what prompted my interest in the village. I replied that my interest was from a mental health perspective. That I was looking for a way to help people live more sustainably by changing the way they thought about their connection with nature. She looked at me and said, "Then you must know of Joanna Macy." I blinked, "Who is Joanna Macy?" She laughed warm-heartedly and said, "Dear, you absolutely have to read her work."

3

Ecopsychology: Finding Ourselves in Nature and Finding Nature in Ourselves

If we surrendered to Earth's intelligence, we could rise up rooted, like trees. Instead, we entangle ourselves in knots of our own making and struggle, lonely and confused.

Rainer Maria Rilke, Austrian poet, and novelist

Joanna Macy, I discovered, is one of the most marvelous pioneering women of our time. She is an author, Buddhist scholar, and environmental activist. Again, if you already know of her work, please feel free to skip or refresh.

Since I knew nothing about her at that time, I dove into her writing and tried to absorb as much of it as I could. Through her I embraced her ideas of Despair and Empowerment Work, now called the Work that Reconnects, which recognizes that for humans to reconnect with their environment they must allow themselves to touch the pain and despair that arises both from our disconnection, as well as our deep understanding that our environment's destruction is real. Our waters are polluted, our air is polluted, our soil is contaminated, our Earth is being fracked and hacked and cemented and burned and mined. It is real. And it really hurts if we let that reality into our hearts, minds, and bodies. Through allowing ourselves to feel the pain rather than numb it, we can be re-empowered to make changes for ourselves and the rest of the natural world we inhabit. This was clearly a "how" that had a track record behind it.

I began taking her ideas into workshops for other clinicians. One bright Los Angeles afternoon I expectantly addressed a group of around 20 mental health professionals. The conference room was small but comfortable. After sharing with each other what brought each of them to the workshop, we went into the experiential part of the day. I asked them to pair up and gave each couple a large container with various natural elements for them to experience and explore — sand, soil, water, rocks, feathers, plants. I used Macy's template to facilitate a felt connection first with themselves, then each other and finally with these natural elements.

In Macy's method, groups of people are guided to open to their connection to nature and specifically to the grief each feels over the condition of the world. Allowing each person to open to, rather than fearing and numbing the feelings that arise, is a crucial step in becoming one with our environment again. When we are in touch with the suffering of animals, destruction of rainforests, pollution of waters and all the other pains humans inflict on our Earthmates, we are moved. And when we are moved, we want to act. Numbing allows stagnancy. Movement creates change.

Many people expressed a deep resonance with the experience. There were tears as well as laughs. Beauty and insight. Hearts and minds opened.

Despite the success, though, I got mixed responses from people about wanting to continue the work. Some were very inspired and wanted to continue while others expressed uncertainty. When I asked them about it, they talked about not wanting to have to experience the pain. As a grief specialist, I understood that our social norms around loss have also gotten very weak. We have barely retained the rituals that help us grieve, much less allow it to enter our daily life. Our civilized culture promotes birth and youthfulness, acquisition and accumulation and eternal bliss as signs of success. Loss and pain are seen as failure, pain being something that should be denied, avoided, numbed, or hidden.

I found that a good number of clinicians, as well as lay people, though acknowledging the pain, wanted a method that would allow them to feel uplifted and hopeful. Although I wasn't sure what that might look like, I accepted that delving into the depths of shared psychic pain as our environment is destroyed could be overwhelming. This may be especially true post-pandemic, as our climate crisis clock is running out. It occurred to me that to hit the mainstream with despair work might be too challenging and would take more time than I thought was prudent. I deeply believe in and recommend Macy's work wholeheartedly. I recently had the privilege of being in conversation with her. At 94, she is as bold and inspiring as ever in her encouragement and conviction that as ordinary people we have the power to shift the direction we are headed in, if we have the courage to face reality and choose love of life over fear. If you feel yourself drawn to her practices, and have the support around the inevitable grief, please do them. All ecotherapy methods are mutually supportive of each other and it is always essential for us to have ways to connect with the reality of our global crisis if we are to reclaim our natural mind.

With the realization that many people are underprepared to touch the magnitude of this pain, I knew I would have to keep searching for the method of change I wanted to facilitate. I continued my personal practices of mindfulness meditation, sensory connection in nature, and an unwavering commitment to finding anyone and everyone that had a similar interest in ecopsychology. I knew there must be someone that had developed a structured, proven way of helping people shift their consciousness around nature that I was looking for. I just had to keep practicing and keep searching. It would be another 11 years before I found that someone and that answer.

Reflection Invitation

I invite you to notice what comes up for you when you consider opening yourself to the pain and despair of our current relationship with and destruction of the rest of nature? If you feel drawn to experience Joanna Macy's practices, please visit her website (www.joannamacy.net) for resources.

The idea of surrendering to Earth's intelligence as Rilke advises in his quote at the beginning of this chapter seems to pose a threat to our human ego. The modern human psyche demonstrates how threatening an idea it is to see ourselves as part of a whole "web of interbeing" by its insistence on separating itself out. This is true in modern Western psychology as well, and almost always goes unexamined and unaddressed.

The premise of approaching mental health from a standpoint of "humans as Earth" operates in alignment with the premise that people cannot be well until we are thinking, feeling, and behaving in harmony again with what I call our Earthbody. I want to emphasize again that your own definitions and unfolding understanding of your relationship to your planet is primary. That said, I will share my thoughts on what Earthbody means to me at this point.

Think of it this way: humans are to their Earthbody as kidneys are to their human body. Our kidneys are an organ with a particular purpose for our whole human body, but it doesn't exist or function without the whole body, nor is it more, or less, important than the other parts, for example our skin. Similarly, humans are a species with a particular purpose for our Earthbody, but we don't exist outside our Earthbody, nor are we more important than the other parts, for example our soil. Although our kidneys are unique, the idea that they are "separate from" our skin or our entire body is false. Similarly, although humans are unique, the idea that we are "separate from" our soil or our entire planet is equally false.

And again, even if we *think* we are separate, we can't be.

Reflection Invitation

I invite you to take a moment right now to reflect on how you see *yourself* in relationship to *your* Earthbody. What does that language bring up in your mind? Do you notice any judgment? Any confusion? What does "Earthbody" mean? Do you sense yourself *as* the Earth or *on* the Earth? All answers are fine, even a sense of confusion, it's simply an important step to notice how you perceive yourself in relation to the rest of nature.

To go even further with the idea that separation is an illusion, we can look to chemistry. We have all come to accept that matter, things we can touch, like tables, chairs, air, water, trees — even humans — are all made up of molecules. We also agree that molecules are made up of atoms, and that atoms in part are made of even tinier parts called electrons. Electrons are all the same no matter which element they're creating. So, on the sub-particle level, the electrons in your body "touch" the electrons in the air, the air's electrons "touching" the electrons in the floor. There is no separation. And if you really want to blow your mind, you can let yourself realize that not only is our entire planet connected in this tapestry of electrons, but the space around Earth, our moon, other planets, the stars, our entire galaxy and all the known and unknown galaxies are unified this way. Endlessly. But for now, let's just stick to the bond between humans and the rest of Earth.

Let's consider ecosystems. Put simply, an ecosystem is a community of living organisms in a particular area that are linked together through nutrient and energy flows and interacting as a system. Sometimes we call this a "food chain" or "food web." Almost all these systems have been studied and put together *without including humans*. Interesting.

Pioneering the inclusion of humans in various ecosystems, ecologist and complex systems scientist, Jennifer Dunne, of the Santa Fe Institute is leading a project with archaeologist, Stefani Crabtree, of the Santa Fe Institute and Center for Research and Interdisciplinarity. One of their studies examines the role of Australian Aboriginal people. The Martu are a group of five distinct Indigenous tribal groups in the Western Desert of Australia. Martu are hunter-gatherers and live in small groups of less than 100 members. They are an egalitarian system; both men and women hunt for food which is shared with all members. Food sharing is a source of prestige although prestige is not the motivation for food sharing.

According to Crabtree, Martu Aboriginal foragers stabilized their ecosystem by providing several ecosystem services such as lighting small brush fires to expose the burrows of small prey. The scorched patches left on the landscape served as natural fire breaks against larger, more devastating wildfires. When the Martu were removed from their homeland in the mid-twentieth century, wildfires increased dramatically in size, and several small mammals, like the Rufous hare-wallaby, became extinct in that area (Santa Fe Institute, February 18, 2019). This serves as only one example of how nature embedded humans play a role in the sustainability of an ecosystem within which they believe themselves to be, and function as, a part of the whole.

What might our modern life be like if we all saw ourselves as part of a larger web of life? I'd like to take a moment to hypothesize that since we have been functioning for so long in a culture that uses separation, domination, and oppression, we have simply forgotten our role in our ecosystem. Perhaps our role would reemerge effortlessly. Again, I'm not suggesting that we return to the jungle. Rather I invite you to consider that a nature embedded way of life may actually be more comfortable and less stressful for us and that when we repair our natural bond we will remember and reclaim more physical and emotional health overall. I also believe that as we reintegrate our natural relationship with our environment, a new culture will evolve that includes technology, but prizes a more holistic life-sustaining way of behaving. We are beginning to bring concepts like "People over Profit" into our discussion of social values. Similarly, a culture that values the entire planetary web of inter-beings might operate as "Planet over Profit." Again, with the understanding that *people* and *planet* are one and the same, there is no Being left unaccounted for.

At this point, given the state people are in with each other, you may be wondering if we might need to repair our human bonds before we can leap to repairing our nature bond and caring about all beings. This question is understandable. It does seem like that repair would need to be addressed first. I'll go into more detail in later parts of this book, but in brief, our human-to-human bonds are also healed through the ANFT-style of nature therapy I will introduce you to in Chapter Four. One of the most healing aspects of this model is its group format and Circle practice as the way of processing, integrating, and deepening one's experience. In Circle practice the group takes turns speaking in the moment from their hearts about what they are experiencing. This is not a typical conversation but rather a way for each person to speak and be listened to without interruption. Using the process of Circle shares between invitations creates a space where every voice is equally valued to process the group's shared experience. Each individual share is seen as an important ingredient in the whole group's integrated perspective — as if the group was an entity with multiple heads, all adding the perspectives the whole group needs to hear. Most people leave these nature immersions with a sense of being more relaxed and bonded with the other people in the group in a very uncommon way. The groups begin as strangers, but in a few hours end with a sense of true connection with the land as well as the people. Although nature immersions can be done alone, the group experience is a crucial component in healing our human relational wounds caused by a cultural system of competition and domination. Using this model, we heal our human relations as we build and repair our relationship to our planetary relations.

The epidemic psychosis of our time is the lie of believing we have no ethical obligation to our planetary home. —Theodore Roszak, American historian, author, scholar, pacifist, teacher, and social critic

Theodore Roszak was born in my hometown of Chicago. Credited with coining the term Ecopsychology, he advocated for the need for humans to reconnect with nature as the path to individual and cultural sanity. Here are his words (1995):

"Ecopsychology has a greater cultural project: to redefine the relationship of the natural environment to sanity in our time. Ecotherapists wish to heal the soul while engaging the whole. We wish to speak for the planet and its imperiled species. We wish to recall the long-forgotten Anima Mundi and honor it in our relations and work. We wish to converse with primary people to foster healing and build common cause. The planetary environment is the context for healing the soul because the two are inextricably bound by bonds that are sacred: life and consciousness. Implicit in this project is the need for a scientific paradigm that gives life and consciousness a new central status in the universe. Based upon such a paradigm, ecopsychology is more than a mere academic exercise; it is part of an ongoing and practical healing mission that recognizes and honors that the health of the individual human psyche depends upon the collective health of all the kingdoms of life on Earth."

From this paradigm, sanity or mental health and insanity or mental illness must be defined in relationship to the rest of nature. Or put another way, our self-identity must be connected not just to our individual body, or our societal body, but must expand out to our Earthbody; meaning that we perceive our natural environment as our self. For example, the orange tree in my front yard and I are one. The tree is the part of me that grows out of the soil producing oranges and emitting oxygen into the air, and I am the part of the tree that takes in the oxygen, eats the fruit, perhaps spreading the seeds to other locations as I move around emitting carbon dioxide into the air that the tree takes in.

And perhaps a final definition of "sane" is life-sustaining, and "insane" is life-threatening. Human behaviors and actions that sustain human, animal, plant, and planetary life are sane and those that threaten those lives are insane.

To that end, Ecopsychology puts forth the following three precepts outlined here by John Davis, Ph.D. (Naropa University and School of Lost Borders, October 2006):

1. There is a deeply bonded and reciprocal relationship between humans and nature. Ecopsychology draws on two metaphors for this relationship: nature as home and family (e.g., Earth as mother, animals as siblings) and nature as Self, in which self-identifications are broadened to include the "greater-than-human" world and Gaia.

2. The illusion of a separation of humans and nature leads to suffering both for the environment (as ecological devastation) and for humans (as grief, despair, and alienation).

3. Realizing the connection between humans and nature is healing for both. This reconnection includes the healing potential of contact with nature, work on grief and despair about environmental destruction, ecotherapy, and psycho-emotional bonding with the world as a source of environmental action and sustainable lifestyles. A specifically ecopsychological approach would include both the psychological and the environmental in such reconnection. It is this inclusion of both the "eco" and the "psyche" which distinguishes ecopsychology from both environmentalism and psychology.

A thought about the first precept — I believe both metaphors are useful; the latter being much more challenging than the former. It is my hope that we will, as a species, attain a state of heart and mind where we self-identify with each other and the "greater-than-human" world. I believe living with a sense of oneness with the planet is an evolutionary shift. That said, making the first shift that recognizes and respects all living beings as equal in value is pivotal and perhaps is the only gateway to being able to fully identify with the whole. After all, if we've spent enough time living with a perspective of respect for other species it might be easier to want to identify with them as ourselves.

The last precept is important and needs a bit of clarification. Historically environmentalists have focused on the concern about, and actions aimed at, protecting our natural world with the field of psychology focusing only on human behavior and mind. By including both "eco" and "psyche" we define a paradigm that reunifies the two parts of one whole. Mending the artificial split.

I would also like to add to Dr Davis' list of how this split hurts the environment by raising the possibility that this human illusion of separation from nature may also lead to another kind of suffering for the environment, in addition to the observable ecological devastation Dr Davis mentions. I would like to invite the idea that the greater-than-human world might experience having "lost" us. There is no reason to believe that it isn't possible for other beings to have some sense about our lost connection. This kind of thought rests on a foundational premise that allows other beings to have intelligence and awareness and, therefore, an awareness of our species. Though it may not be identical to our human form of experiencing loss, might it be possible that we are missed? If one does want to consider this possibility, it might follow that our fellow Earthmates may attempt to reach out to us for reconnection. It may be easier to recognize and accept this idea by thinking about how a beloved cat or dog invites us to connect with them when they miss our attention. As I am writing this paragraph, my cat has jumped up on the back of my chair and is rubbing his face against my head. Might other beings, trees, plants, rivers, also draw our attention to them in recognizable ways if we look for it?

Reflection Invitation

I invite you to imagine what it might look like if the rest of nature feels our disconnection. Can you imagine how your environment might seek to reach out to you? For example, might a flower attract you by its fragrance? If you'd like, go outside with this idea in mind ... do you notice any ways that the more-than-human beings attract your attention? Journal about your experience if you like.

Although I truly believe that contemplating and experiencing our emotional connection with the rest of nature is the way to understanding the importance of our bond, having scientific evidence regarding the benefit of our human-nature connection brings the conversation to a concrete level. It gives us the safety and security most of us need to step outside our perceptual cage without risk of humiliation and social exile. No matter how much we may love the idea of reconnecting with nature and shifting back to a sustainable egalitarian paradigm that respects all the Earth's elements, none of us wants to risk being labeled as "weird," "woo-woo," or "crunchy." With that in mind, let's look at what science has found.

Current research on the neuroscience of nature is exploding exponentially as we discover from the inside out not only *that* humans are optimized in connection with the natural world, but *how*. Meaning that nature connection has proven benefits to humans physically, cognitively, and emotionally. To put it simply, we function much better in green settings than we do in urban or digital settings. Even simply looking at a photo of a natural setting will begin to change our physiology and mood in positive ways. Spending non-goal-oriented time outdoors in sensory connection with the rest of nature improves our bodies, our minds, and the way we behave.

To tell the story of the scientific exploration of the human-nature connection and the benefits of Forest Bathing (Shinrin Yoku) and Forest therapy in particular, we must travel back in time to Japan in 1982. Due to the shift to a technology-based economy, the population saw steep increases in sub-health conditions such as chronic fatigue, forgetfulness, dizziness, back soreness, poor appetite, depression, congestion, proneness to colds and flu, and general body weakness to name a few as well as lifestyle diseases such as diabetes, heart disease, hypertension, and some forms of cancer. At that time, the director of Japan's Forest Agency, Tomohide Akiyama, coined the term Shinrin Yoku (Forest Bathing) to encourage people to bathe in the atmosphere of the forests both to improve their own health and to create a desire to protect the country's ancient forest land. Japan is home to amazing old-growth forests with many trees over 1000 years old. It was Akiyama's intent to make sure Japan maintained a natural desire to protect them.

Although Akiyama's Shinrin Yoku was based on common sense, ten years later, Dr Yoshifumi Miyazaki of Chiba University conducted the first scientific study to show the measurable beneficial effects of spending time (40 minutes of walking) in the forests versus the same amount of time and activity in a laboratory. His was the first of many future published studies from Chiba University as well as studies from a separate group from Kyoto that demonstrate actual changes in cortisol levels, blood pressure, heart rate and mood in the people spending time in nature versus their counterparts indoors. This collection of published research confirmed that spending unstructured time in a forest setting reduces psychological stress, depression, anxiety, hostility and improves mental ability, sleep, mood, and a sense of aliveness. That was only the beginning.

By 2019, a total of five countries or regions—Japan, South Korea, Poland, China, and Taiwan—have conducted empirical studies on the health effects of Forest Bathing (Shinrin Yoku) and it doesn't seem to be stopping.

In their book *Your Brain on Nature: The Science of Nature's Influence on Your Health, Happiness, and Vitality* (2012), authors Eva M. Selhub, MD and Alan C. Logan, ND, report a vast number of ways humans benefit in nature from cognitive improvement, boosts in the immune system, improved mood and lowered destructive stress hormones. They reference the work of Erich Fromm, a German American psychoanalyst, and Edward O. Wilson, an American biologist, as two proponents of the idea that humans are hard-wired to love and affiliate with nature and other life forms, a concept referred to as biophilia. Biophilia is an innate emotional affinity that human beings have for other living organisms. It's in our DNA.

Continuing to explore studies of the human-nature connection in the field of psychology brings us to a fascinating understanding of the modern problem of attention fatigue. Harvard psychologist, William James, distinguished two forms of attention: voluntary and involuntary. Voluntary attention requires intentional sustained effort to focus on the task and ignore distractions. Mental fatigue was explained as the stress and fatigue that builds up as we spend prolonged periods of time using focused attention. Involuntary attention, by contrast, is an effortless process where there is a degree of interest or excitement as the motivation. Oftentimes, involuntary attention feels like an organic meandering of the attention guided by a sense of pleasure or fascination. Involuntary attention is effortless and allows the mind to make fresh and surprising connections between things, which results in less fatigue. In the late 1970's, Dr Stephen Kaplan advanced this theory and proposed that nature itself might provide the reset button for the mentally fatigued mind.

"Kaplan formalized the initial cognitive-nature theory as Attention Restoration Theory (ART), with four major components proposed for the cognitively restorative environment:

Being Away

This may be physically going somewhere away from the task, but it can also simply refer to breaking the focused attention and letting the mind wander or imagine.

Fascination

The environment should provide the experience of 'soft' fascination (like watching ocean waves) rather than 'hard' fascination (like watching a sporting event).

Extent

The environment must provide considerable depth in order to engage the mind significantly. For example, wandering through a meadow.

Compatibility

The environment provides a way of fulfilling the individual's intentions without struggle and effort. Even a brief visit to a park will most likely meet the individual's expectations.

Kaplan proposed that we might be able to remedy the negative effects of too much focused attention and the attention fatigue it creates by taking advantage of natural settings." (Selhub, Logan 2012,64–65)

These are just a small sample of the findings that abound regarding the physical benefits, mental benefits and emotional benefits nature has to offer. Sound compelling? Ready to jump on board? Probably. But wait. I feel called to remind us that all these studies, while extremely valuable and important in validating how and why humans do so well when we're connected to the rest of nature, were developed from within "the cage," so to speak. The maladaptive cognitive premise that humans are separate from, superior to, and can, therefore, feel free to use nature as a means to human ends, is embedded in the language and structure of this research.

I want to invite you to check with yourself right now to see if you are falling for the idea that nature is a fantastic medicine for us to use for our physical and mental ailments. If so, see if you can shift to a more adaptive nature embedded premise that when we are in a reciprocal relationship with the rest of our Earthmates, we feel, think, and act differently. *Naturally,* we are kinder, gentler, healthier, more creative beings when we reclaim our place in our ecological family. *Naturally,* we are kinder, gentler, healthier, more creative beings when we are embedded in our Earthbody. No being needs to use any other being for their own personal gain.

On that note, I'd like to bring attention to the work of Clemens G. Arvay. Arvay was an Austrian-born plant biologist and non-fiction author whose books emphasize health ecology. Two of his most important works in terms of human connection with the rest of nature are *The Biophilia Effect* (2018) and *The Healing Code of Nature* (2018). I believe a crucial element of his work is his emphasis that this is a connection, a bond *between* beings. There is a natural relationship that consists of an ongoing flow of communication between humans and the other-than-human beings we live with. Whether we are aware of it or not, humans are in constant communication with the other beings we encounter. For example, "Plants communicate directly with our immune system and (our) unconscious without us even needing to touch, much less swallow, them... Plants heal without having to be processed into teas, creams, essences, extracts, oils, perfumes, or drops and tablets. They heal us through biological communication that our immune system and unconscious mind understand" (Arvay, 2018, 5).

Communication is defined as the transmission of information between a sender and a receiver. How this information is coded is critical in understanding interspecies communication. In the case of plants, the information is coded in terpenes (chemical substances created and emitted for various interactions). Insects also use chemical substances. And so do we. Not only do plants emit these substances, but they do them intentionally in response to environmental conditions. For example, you, sitting under a pine tree. As you rest against this loving being, kicking your shoes off and gazing up at her branches, your immune system is communicating, sending information to her. She receives the information and releases her terpenes and phytoncides (a compound related to immunity) which you absorb through your lungs and maybe your skin if you've chosen to feel her bark for some reason. After a while, as the two of you converse in this way, the number of natural killer cells in your immune system will increase considerably. Not only will they increase in number, but they will be much more active. And this activity will go on for days. The level of anticancer proteins, with which your immune system prevents or fights cancer with, will also be elevated. Interesting conversation, don't you think? Quite a gift.

And in exchange, you, of course, gifted the tree with your carbon dioxide and nitrogen-filled exhale. If you, as you sat beneath this tree, were consciously aware of this exchange, this communication, is there anything else you might want to communicate to this being? Anything else you might want to give?

With all this evidence of how our human-nature partnership helps us physically and emotionally, you may be feeling yourself beginning to warm up to the idea of including it in your self-care plan and maybe even your clients' treatment plans if you are a helping professional. I would like to offer another gentle reminder. Remember that it is ingrained in our mind that we separate ourselves out and use the rest of nature in service to our single species' needs. It's very tempting to latch on to nature as a commodity. Remember that this premise continues to support an abusive relationship between humans and non-humans, where the latter is still in servitude to the former. Our ideal premise respects all beings and elements as co-inhabitants of our biome or, as stated earlier, our largest self. With a scientific understanding only of how humans are benefited by the rest of nature, we haven't healed the psychic tear that continues to sicken our bodies and minds. We will continue to suffer anxiety, depression, and physical illness.

Continuing to believe that we are separate from Earth is like believing our hand is somehow separate from our body. Or more accurately, that our hand believes itself to be separate because its function is unique from the other parts of the body. It would be ridiculous to try and function from that premise; yet this is how humans relate to the rest of their biosphere. We need to remember that *we are* nature to fully heal ourselves within the rest of nature. To mend our mutual psyche.

Therefore, an understanding of the human benefits of being in nature is only one step closer (albeit a critical step in terms of creating a genuine desire to protect the natural world from human inflicted harm) to the ultimate goal of recognizing the indivisibility between our human selves and the rest of nature. When we recognize this indivisibility, we remember that we are not entitled to dominate or use nature solely for our own gains, and reciprocity enters the conversation. The heartfelt question can arise, "What can I give back to the beings around me?" This perceptual shift is a much bigger leap for most of us. That shift needs therapeutic intervention.

Reflection Invitation

How do you feel about giving back to other beings? Can you imagine ways you can acknowledge what you're receiving and reciprocate in some way? Can you think of at least five ways you can give to the other-than-human beings you encounter each day?

4

Ecotherapy: I Already Spend Time Outdoors, What's the Difference?

When one tugs at a single thing in nature, he finds it attached to the rest of the world.
John Muir, Scottish American naturalist, author, and environmental philosopher

Thankfully, I forgot my book while traveling back from visiting family in Santa Fe to Los Angeles one Tuesday morning in 2016. The flight was short, but long enough for me to decide to read the in-flight magazine cover to cover, and there, between the advertisements for travel pillows and sudoku puzzles, the words "Shinrin Yoku" opened the door to what I had been searching for over the past eleven years. I read through the article which described a practice called "Forest Bathing" developed by M. Amos Clifford. My heart and mind raced like I imagine a miner might feel seeing the glint of a diamond or vein of gold. If this practice proved to be what I thought it was, it would take me clearly into the "how" of healing our split psyche.

As mentioned earlier, Shinrin Yoku prescribes leisurely walks through the forest to combat illnesses related to over-exposure to urban settings. The practice follows a medical model and, depending on the person's ailment, a frequency and location will be recommended. Each forest itself is ranked in terms of how effective its atmosphere is in positively influencing a person's vital signs. Shinrin Yoku is prescribed as a medical intervention in the same way as any other medicine is, with regular doses over time. The article went on to talk about the psychological benefits of the practice as well, and its effectiveness in treating depression and anxiety.

Clifford's model of Forest Bathing was influenced by this Japanese practice, but by integrating it with other practices (wilderness guiding, Zen meditation, psychotherapy, and nature connection), and removing the medical model, he created a framework that was proving to be an effective, user-friendly, standard method that could be used by anyone, anywhere, anytime. In 2012 he founded the Association of Nature and Forest Therapy (ANFT) with the goal of certifying 1000 forest therapy guides in the US and abroad as a new wellness practice.

As the plane landed and the flight attendant announced that cell service was allowed, I was already sending an email to the man interviewed in the article, Ben Page, ANFT's Director of Training. Ben, fortunately for me, also lived in Los Angeles, was a certified guide through ANFT, and a trainer/mentor for other guides. I was thrilled to find that he frequently led forest therapy walks in the Angeles Forest and that I could learn more about this ecotherapy practice and how it might help me accomplish my goal as a mental health professional.

I arrived home very excited. Right here in my hometown was a program, a philosophy that addressed and synthesized the ideas and dreams I'd been looking for and trying to patch together on my own for the last decade. It was almost too good to be true. I quickly registered for Ben's upcoming walk, although almost solely as a formality. I was certain based on what I'd read that this practice would be the answer. I had researched this style of nature therapy and it spoke to me immediately in some important ways.

As I said, the Association of Nature and Forest Therapy is the brainchild of M. Amos Clifford. Clifford synthesized his background in wilderness tracking, Zen Buddhism, and psychotherapy to come up with a user-friendly, standard method of bringing the benefits of what typically takes a week or longer of isolated retreat in nature into an urban-friendly model of two to three hours of small group connection with the rest of nature.

I want to take a moment to recognize that there are many forms of nature therapy developing all over the planet as we seem to be "waking up" to our Earthbody. And I do believe that all forms of human-nature repair are valuable and have a much-needed place in our healing. I would, however, like to focus in this book only on the practice of ANFT-style nature therapy for some important reasons. First, I believe in this model's systematic and standardized approach. All guides are trained and retrained uniformly to lead through invitations that emphasize the relationship between the participant and the rest of nature. Second, I have personally witnessed the immediate shift this model offers to participants without exception. Third, it has been intentionally designed to benefit anyone regardless of age, race, religion, culture, gender, physical or emotional health, or mobility. Fourth, it provides healing and repair regardless of one's current relationship to the rest of nature. I have watched how it works for people who already have an affinity for nature, as well as for people who feel uncomfortable outdoors and away from concrete. And fifth, it provides repair in human-to-human communication at the same time as it fosters human-nature repair.

I also want to re-emphasize that while being in nature, walking, hiking, biking, camping and all the other outdoor activities people may enjoy doing are beneficial, these are not forms of nature therapy. Common outdoor activity is typically goal-oriented. It may be for working out, recreation, or something else, but it is not seen as purely a time for being in relationship with the more-than-human world. Or there may be distractions like thinking, planning, talking with other people, listening to music, eating, drinking, etc. In typical outdoor activity, nature is only the backdrop for something else. Nature therapy highlights developing relationships as its only purpose.

At the end of each immersion I lead, I like to ask participants how this experience compares with their other outdoor activities, if they have them, and how it differs, if it does. I haven't had a single person yet who doesn't make a clear and overwhelming statement that it's completely different. For example, Mary came to one of my monthly Forest Therapy walks at a local trail. It's a trail I affectionately call "Tadpole Creek" where I used to take my daughter looking for tadpoles when she was about 5 or 6 years old. The trail opens off a busy street, but soon begins to quiet down as you walk deeper along the trail, passing tall, evergreen trees toward a small creek that runs through the canyon. Along the trail the usual runners, hikers and families pass each other consistently. Mary mentioned to me that she was an avid hiker and often hiked this same trail that we used for our immersion. I asked her if she found any difference between our immersion and her hikes. She immediately answered, "I come here all the time. In fact, I was here just last weekend. But after this experience I feel like I've never really noticed it before today." Nathan, another participant put it this way, "I was surprised to find that I actually felt a bond with the tree I sat with. Even though it was only twenty minutes. I didn't expect to feel that." It isn't unusual for people to report some kind of unexpected connection with one or more of the more-than-human beings they are invited to interact with — a tree, a stream, blades of grass, a dragonfly, the air, rain. Many times, people express that they experience something surprisingly like a newfound friendship. Or a reawakening to a time in their childhood where these connections were frequent and pleasurable. Keeping in mind that this way is our natural way of being with nature that we have been trained away from, it isn't surprising. Reestablishing this natural bonding is the essential difference that ANFT-style nature and forest therapy helps cultivate.

Reflection Invitation

When you spend time in nature, are you doing something like hiking, biking, or some other goal-oriented sort of activity? When was the last time you were with the rest of nature simply being or observing? Do you remember something like lying on the ground as a child and looking up at the clouds with no other agenda? Would you like to do that now?

5

Defining the Therapist: What Do I Do with My Ego and All the Letters I've Collected after My Name?

Sell your cleverness and buy bewilderment. Cleverness is mere opinion. Bewilderment brings intuitive knowledge.

Rumi, thirteenth century Persian poet,
theologian, and mystic

This chapter addresses mental health and allied professionals who already work with people, as well as people who are interested in becoming forest therapy guides. Guides do not have to be therapists, but I am suggesting that therapists should become certified guides. If you fall into the group of people who don't have an interest in guiding, you may want to read this chapter anyway since it will give you insight into how you might select a therapist, healer, or guide and be able to identify where they are in their own psychological shift.

I've heard some clinicians say that they have plants in their office because they understand that nature has a great healing effect on people. To be blunt, having plants in our office is not ecotherapy for our clients, unless perhaps we put the plant in our coveted chair and step aside to allow them to make a connection with each other.

At a recent Forest Therapy conference, I led a discussion group for mental health professionals with an interest or practice in nature therapy. We met together under a canopy of pine trees, many sitting on the soft dirt or on folded blankets breathing in the fresh air and gazing off at a small lake, a paddling of ducks gliding back and forth nearby. I posed the question to the group, "When we're leading people in a nature therapy experience, who is the therapist, you or the land?" I thought the question was rhetorical and that everyone there would have a shared laugh at the idea that we were the therapist. I assumed the group would agree that Nature was the therapist and the relationship between our clients and the rest of nature was where the healing occurred. I was surprised to hear from at least half the group that they believed they were the therapists and used nature to help their clients. For them nature was another tool in the kit.

I appreciate this mistake and have compassion for those who make it. It's something I had to consciously correct in myself often in the beginning. We are so accustomed to seeing nature as a commodity rather than an equal partner in life as we know it, and so accustomed to seeing ourselves as the authority. However, the reparative answer is that Nature is the therapist. The Association of Nature and Forest Therapy puts it this way, "The Forest is the therapist. The Guide opens the doors." These two simple sentences speak volumes. The forest or the rest of nature is in charge of whatever therapy or healing is needed for the people that we lead in this practice. The guide acts in service to the relationship between Nature and people. The guide takes their cues from Nature.

Reflection Invitation

I invite you to take that into your own heart and mind as well. What does this shift in role bring up for you? Can you imagine yourself stepping aside and only acting as a support for the therapy that occurs between someone and another being (a shrub, a stream, a rock for example)? Can you trust that the healing is between them, with you as the witness and container? Simply notice whatever comes up.

For some mental health professionals, this idea may be very challenging. For some it may bring up confusion. It may even threaten our identity and our ego. As clinicians we have put a lot of time, energy and money into our education, our theoretical orientations, our evidence-based interventions, and in honing our skills to become excellent at our work in helping people move beyond their limits and achieve greater levels of mental, emotional, and relational health. It's no wonder we can be reluctant to give over that role. This is especially true if we haven't repaired our own relationship with the rest of nature enough to fully understand that the more-than-human beings around us are equally able to heal, transform, and communicate. The guide's relationship with the forest is an essential part of how well she, he or they will be able to step out of the conventional role as healer, teacher, or therapist.

As we repair our own relationship with the land, two areas come forward in importance: how the guide spends time with Nature and how the guide learns to craft invitations based on the land. Similarly to becoming a skilled clinician, our personal healing is essential in making the necessary shift to truly be able to facilitate another person's healing. Again, we can only take people as far as we've gone ourselves. This is why I believe the kind of guide certification ANFT provides is such an important distinction. I will go into more detail about the certification process through ANFT and share my own experience with it in the next chapter.

How the guide spends time with Nature and how often, is probably the most influential aspect of authentically making this paradigm shift. The ANFT certification process includes a six-month practicum following the initial eight-day immersive training. During this mentored practicum, guides spend each day in communion with the land. Sitting, observing, drawing, encountering the more-than-human world on their own, as well as leading people to connect with local trails and collecting feedback from participants on what their experience was like during the walk. Additionally, there are reading and writing assignments that continue fostering the guide's relationship with nature.

If left unaddressed, our own unhealed relationship (most importantly our ability to step out of the "therapist" or "healer" role) may create an obstacle to stepping into the vital role of supporting the relationship between our clients and the other beings around them. Our ego may interfere with this bond, rather than fostering it. One example of how this might happen is how an invitation is designed. An invitation that predicts or tries to manipulate how the participant should experience their relationship with another being is an indication that the guide is taking the wrong role. If the guide sets up an expectation that something specific should occur, "Find a tree that makes you feel happy," it disregards and disrespects the organic relationship between the two beings, whatever condition that relationship is currently in. When the guide steps out of the way, however, and lets the forest be the therapist, "Find a tree and spend twenty minutes with it. What do you notice?" the participant is free to notice what occurs between themself and the tree, including nothing at all. This approach gives full respect to the relationship between the participant and the tree, allowing whatever arises or doesn't arise to be accepted as "right." In turn, this cultivates a sense of trust in the participant and the beings they interact with. Teaching the person to trust their own reactions without judgment, even in cases that feel "negative," is essential.

If we continue to cling to our identity as a therapist or healer and take the position that *we* are responsible for a therapeutic intervention, it's indicative of that faulty premise, the conceptual cage, that separates us out from the whole rest of nature. And unfortunately, it also perpetuates placing ourselves at the top of an unhealthy imaginary hierarchy. Humans as the "top of the food chain."

Shifting our perception to *partnering* with the rest of nature is crucial to the kind of healing I'm talking about. Without it we are only making half the step we need to make. And we will not ultimately heal the psychic tear that creates the ills we are intending to correct.

Reflection Invitation

I invite you to reflect for a moment right now on the effect it has inside you when you consider yourself as a partner with the land, as a guide opening the door for people to make connection with the Forest as the therapist. What do you notice shifts inside you? Do you sense any resistance to giving over the locus of healing to the land instead of yourself?

Giving the role of therapist over to the land itself may challenge our sense of control. In truth, we have no idea what may occur between someone and the land or what condition their relationship is in, if they have one at all. It can be very tempting to want to provide a "good" outcome. It can be tempting to have people feel a certain way with the land. But again, this disrespects the actual relationship and won't allow that relationship to go through what it needs to heal. If you can imagine providing therapy with a parent and child where you spent the session trying to make them feel a certain way toward each other, you might begin to understand how equally non-therapeutic that approach is with any human-nature relationship.

Once we begin to trust the natural world, we can let go of trying to control the outcome. We can trust that whatever someone experiences is correct and corrective. Even when it looks negative.

Anita and Susan were two sisters that expressed an interest in the practice of ANFT-style forest bathing. Anita had recently moved to Los Angeles and was getting her career as a physical therapist going. She was really enjoying the California lifestyle — hiking, biking, yoga, and the ocean. Susan, a CPA, was visiting from their home in Brooklyn. She liked being outdoors but made it clear that she was a "city girl" and didn't go in for the new "woo-woo" activities Anita had been sharing with her lately. Anita looked at me and rolled her eyes, "If she would just let go of being such a control freak, I think she would find such peace in nature. I know I have," her voice trailed off. If I took the bait of being the therapist or healer, I may begin to feel pressure to provide a specific outcome that would make Anita feel validated or show Susan how the practice was not woo-woo or any of the other agendas each of them may have expressed. As a guide, however, my role is to show omnipartiality to what each person is genuinely experiencing in their relationship with nature. Which means caring for and favoring all views and experiences. Anita's deepening bond with the land and Susan's experience of it as woo-woo were both "right." It is not my role to disagree, agree, change, or enhance anyone's experience. That is the role of the land, and it may or may not happen.

I have had more than a few people who haven't "connected" with the land, or who felt it was "too woo-woo" for them. These same folks also said they felt calmer or more energetic at the end of the experience. It's not my business to try and make someone form a particular conclusion about their experience or have a certain relationship with the rest of nature. It's between the two of them to find each other the way they do.

When we let go of trying to manipulate a desired experience or outcome, then we can truly support healing. Watching the repair of this intrinsic bond is fascinating, beautiful and life affirming.

Reflection Invitation

What does omnipartiality mean to you? Do you see it operating in your life now in some way? What do you notice is the felt sense of being omnipartial versus being impartial? What do you notice when you suspend all judgment and desire to create a certain outcome?

6

The Role of the Guide: If the Forest Is the Therapist, Why Do People Need Me There at All?

Liminality lies between the known and the unknown ...
It is a space of heightened intensity that we experience
when we traverse the threshold of the creative unknown.

Anonymous

Nine months after my first Forest Bathing walk on a rugged trail in Monrovia Canyon, I found myself driving up to Northern California to Sugarloaf Ridge State Park. I was about to embark on my own training and certification with ANFT. It was the first training available that I could reasonably get to, as most of the others were out of state or international. My application to become a guide had been approved, I had saved up for the cost of the training, and I had the good fortune to be training with Ben. It gave me some sense of security knowing he would be there. I knew no one else and it eased my mind to know there would be one familiar face.

Everything seemed to be lining up like a clean shot on the 8-Ball. I was anxious, excited, frightened, certain, and completely uncertain all rolled into one. I was stepping way outside my comfort zone, about to tent camp on my own for an intensive eight days with a group of strangers. I had never pitched a tent before, had borrowed the gear from a friend, packed as well as I could, had my journal and recommended reading as well as bringing a photo of my mom with me to encourage me. She had been gone for a long time, but I felt her presence beside me as I leaned into this unknown. My daughter Marley, then 21, had been incredibly supportive to me, encouraging me to go all in to this scary experience, and dear friends confirmed how right this adventure would be for me. I felt it too.

The drive up north from Los Angeles was long, and I thought it would be best to find a place to stay for the night and finish the drive in the morning so that I could start fresh. As I sat alone in my hotel room, the sky grew darker and the streetlamps in the parking lot outside my hotel window cast a dull orange hue. I took my last hot shower, crawled into the pillow topped bed and felt all my domestication wrapping itself around me like a security blanket. How would I do this? Who were these people? What if I was wrong? A voice deeper inside me pushed me on. Whatever lay ahead, I knew it was the answer to something. I secured myself in trusting that voice, glanced at the photo of my mom, turned off the table lamp and fell asleep.

The next morning, I rose early. The sun sparkled on the hood of my car. The air was crisper than I was used to and already smelled of pine. I opened the car windows, turned off the radio and listened to the tires against the asphalt as I headed toward the campground. The directions were confusing as the freeway turned to one lane country roads. I had planned to find a store to get food for myself to last the next eight days. I finally found a small general store and bought what I could. Carrots, hummus, pita bread, oatmeal, nuts, water, apples, peanut butter. I felt like a 10-year-old trying to come up with food that would keep for a week without refrigeration, that I didn't have to cook, and would provide some nutrition. I threw in a box of Earl Grey Tea. I have no idea why, other than it symbolized familiarity. I hoped for the best, put the bag of food in my trunk and headed back to the road. I felt inadequate, guilty for not knowing how to do this, and offered myself the only bit of compassion I could, "It's okay, Julie. Trust."

I turned off the road and entered the campground, winding slowly around to find the site where our group would be for the next eight days. The grounds were surrounded by tall pine trees and mountains, the ground covered with lush grass on one side and a soft golden meadow on the other. It was distinctly Northern California where rain wasn't a stranger, like it is in Los Angeles. The sky even had clouds decorating its familiar blue.

I pulled into the campsite marked "Association of Nature and Forest Therapy" and parked my sedan next to a Jeep where an earthy looking young man was whittling a stick. Tents were being set up in the background, everyone looking as if they'd been doing this kind of thing their whole lives. I offered a weak smile to the whittling man as he offhandedly nodded toward me and I thought, "What the hell am I doing here?"

I saw a table set up where it looked like I could check in. I decided to do that before attempting to touch any of the gear in my trunk. A young person nicknamed Rocket checked me in. They were open and friendly, and though I still felt awkward and apprehensive, the warmth of their personality allowed me to breathe a little. "I've never pitched a tent before. I'm hoping there's someone that can help me," I said half asking and half just putting that reality out there. A woman sitting nearby casually replied, "I'll help you." My first friend.

I handed Rocket my paperwork, releases for injury and the like, and they told me to choose anywhere I liked to set up my tent. I looked around. The land was flat and filled with trees and flowers. On the other side of the campsite was a stream. I thought to myself, "I have no idea what a good spot is. But the water sounds pretty and there are three trees near the bank." I felt drawn to them, like guardians over what would be my place of refuge for the week. I clumsily dragged my things over to the trees, cleared away sticks and stones the way I imagined I should since I would be lying on this "floor" and started to unpack the tent. There was a sweet fragrance in the air. I had never smelled it before. The perfume created a sense of comfort mixed with adventure. Sarah, the woman who was helping me, had a solid, easy presence about her. She calmly told me what to do to pitch my tent. Laughing at my own ignorance as I fumbled with poles and loops and spikes sinking into the soft earth, helped me the way honesty usually does. I was giving myself full permission to not have to know what I was doing, and to not have to hide it. In no time, the tent was up. I thanked Sarah for her help, truly grateful for her aid. I couldn't have done it without her, which in my normal life is rarely true. I live in a familiar routine world where I'm largely capable not only for myself, but for the people around me. As with many of us in the helping profession, I'm self-sufficient. And as Americans, a sign of our successful adulthood is to be able to accomplish a lot on our own. Feeling my need for Sarah's help and her willingness to give it to me was different in a good way.

As she walked away toward her own tent nearby, I turned my attention to the inside of mine. I unzipped the "front door" making sure to quickly zip it again behind me before any mosquitos could enter. The tent was designed to hold four people. With just me inside, I felt the luxury of this inner space. Six thin panels of blue nylon separated me from what now had become "outside." I felt a tiny thrill, like being a child again, hidden in a secret space created by chairs, blankets, and pillows … where the wild things are … ghost stories … flashlights, whispers, and laughter. I unzipped the "windows" of the tent so that I could see the trees beside me. I laid down on my air mattress and looked up through the netting at the canopy of leaves above my head. I felt safer. The sunshine warmed the air. I could hear everyone outside. I took out the photo of my mother and set it up on a stack of books, my journal next to it. My cellphone was useless, no signal, no outlets. I tossed it into my open suitcase of clothes with a feeling of liberation. I tucked my bag of food into another corner and pulled out an apple. "My kitchen," I joked to myself, witnessing my need for order and organization. Everything had its place. I had made my home. I took a deep breath, looked up at the leaves again and felt like a me that I was ready to get to know better. An untamed me.

Reflection Invitation

Find a quiet spot in nature. Let your mind wander and wonder — how do you imagine your "untamed" self?

In a few minutes, I heard a voice outside my tent letting everyone know that our first official Circle would begin in 15 minutes. I zipped my way back out into the open air and brought my camp chair and notebook to the large circle where everyone was gathering. I saw Ben sitting and went over to say hello. He stood up and we hugged, "Hey! Glad you made it!" he smiled. A friendly face, and though we'd only met once before, in that moment, Ben became a kind of anchor for me. "Yes! I'm glad I made it too. This place is beautiful. And there's a fragrance I've never smelled before... Do you know what it is? Where is it coming from?" I asked. "I don't know. I wonder how you might find out...," he smiled. My training had begun.

In the months and years ahead there would be many more lessons like that first one, in understanding the way of the guide. Learning to hold a space in which a person can feel held in liminality by you, yet totally free to explore and expand into their very personal and unique relationship to the natural world, the rest of nature, their Earthbody. Each question that arises in the forest is the forest beckoning. It's Earth starting a conversation that, if answered by the guide, would be a missed opportunity for a relationship to begin and/or deepen. From this perspective, one way to look at my noticing and enjoying the fragrance in the air was the tree starting a conversation with me through its fragrance. It drew me in and made me curious. If Ben had answered me, it would have strengthened our human bond, our friendship, but would have simultaneously weakened, perhaps even blocked, my human-nature bond; my friendship with the tree whose leaves I came to love.

Reflection Invitation

Wander out into your favorite outdoor place — perhaps your yard, a park, a beach. As you move through your environment, notice if you feel curious about something you encounter. Is there a way you can gain some understanding without using a human source, like another person or searching online for an answer to your question?

Our circle was large and spread out beneath the tall California bay laurel trees. In the center of the circle a colorful round cloth covered the ground. There was a candle in the center surrounded by a pine cone, a rock, a small branch, a feather, and a large green leaf. A "talking piece," in this case a large black and white rock, would facilitate our introducing ourselves to each other and setting our intention for ourselves for the week. The group was about 25 people in total, including our trainers and their assistant. We varied in age, gender, orientation, race, religion, nationality, career... with one thing that bound us together: a deep love of the natural world and an intense calling to become a guide. Each of us had a story of what it took to get here, the events that led us to take this journey. For many the decision followed or caused some kind of personal crisis. Every one of us overcame some hardship to be there. It was a bit eerie and comforting all at once. As the talking piece arrived in my hands, I started to speak. Heart racing, not exactly sure if I was making sense, I spoke about the 11 years it took for me to find this path ... my feeling of domestication ... and the burning need to reclaim my personal wilderness ... it felt like a duty, a calling, a way of being I needed beyond logic ... my voice shook, tears flowed. This would not be the only time my heart would break open in the safety of the circle...

What follows next is an account of the training from two perspectives: the trainer and the trainee. The interview gives a behind the scenes insight into the methodology, how the container is created and held, while my journal entries capture my raw transformational process in real time as it unfolded. I want to point out two things. First, a reminder that this account is in no way a training manual. Second, this is an account of my cohort's training. Although there is a solid foundation to what is taught, each cohort brings the coursework to life uniquely, and the coursework has evolved over time to address the Earth's current needs. This is why I believe the initial training is just the beginning of truly understanding this method and regular continuing coursework is highly recommended.

Welcome to Cohort 16:

Ben Page, ANFT trainer/mentor:
The first two days are about building a container that is a safe learning environment. There's a lot of setting the stage for the entire week, and it all begins with this sense of hospitality. For people to learn effectively, they have to feel safe. If they don't feel safe and if they don't understand who they're with and what the group dynamic is, then there's not going to be a very productive learning arc. The learning is so vulnerable. And it's so intense. It's like this kind of deepening spiral. It's

good to just start with that solid foundation. I call it Sunshine and Rainbows Day because we take people out on their first walk and, generally speaking, everyone's just really gaga about their experience and they're just like, "Oh my God, that was so amazing!" But the other thing that goes along with the Sunshine and Rainbows is the way they perceive the actions of the guide. It looks very simple on the surface. People tend to think, "Oh, yeah, so they said some things, and served some tea and, you know, how hard is this really going to be?"

At the end of the day, after our classwork had begun and ended, after I had eaten my dinner and exchanged thoughts with the others, I felt the urge to retreat into the solitude of my tent. Inside, I welcomed the privacy, although the nylon of our tents didn't really create much of a sound barrier. The sun had gone down long ago, and the human night owls continued to talk in the community tent. I awkwardly changed into my pajamas and re-inflated the air mattress. My tent was lit with a small flashlight I had hung above me. I took out another small book light, opened my journal and wrote the first entry:

9:07 p.m. — Journal Entry: First Night
It scares me to be alone in the woods. Even the insects scare me. It scares me to be without my bed — to be so close to the ground. The sticks under me scare me. I feel like this whole forest could hurt me — the plants, the insects, the ground, the rocks, the heat. The people scare me. The "like-minded" people. They seem foreign and dangerous — in what way I have absolutely no idea. How will I possibly sleep? Everything and everyone are strange and unfamiliar and so I am also strange and maybe unfamiliar to myself. I feel myself wanting to make that into a positive. An "opportunity." But I set my intention for this week to be open to my inner self, to open myself up and let in the truth. So, I am trying to connect with the truth. I had no idea how far from the truth I feel. So far, I don't even know how I will recognize

it. I am so accustomed to saying the right and appropriate thing. I don't even know what <u>Truth</u> feels like anymore. But I do know it is truthfully hot in here. I am truthfully afraid and uncomfortable and trying to find any way out of that truth. But I will stay — and see what the truth provides.

In the morning, I woke up early. Across the small meadow was a building with showers and toilets. I decided to venture out into the morning air, use the facilities and take the grounds in on my own. Before breakfast and our training began again, I wrote another entry in my journal. These morning and evening entries were to become my touchstones.

6:47 a.m. — Journal Entry: First Morning

I slept. And it was comfortable. I didn't have any trouble once I had surrendered to sleep the first time — the night and my body carried me through easily. It was cold at some point finally, but all I needed was to wrap the comforter underneath me up around my body and I felt cozy enough to fall back to sleep.

When I finally woke, I was tempted to simply lie in "bed" and listen — which I did do, but then thought better that I go out to the bathroom — my bladder did such a good job for me all night so that I didn't have to find the bathroom in the dark wilderness. I thought after that, I will still have time to come back to "bed" and listen before I join the group. I put on sweats and the sweater I borrowed from Marley and opened the tent to the world again. It was all quiet — I should say peaceful — quiet I guess in the human sense with no one else stirring — the sounds were only the woods. And it was beautiful. I felt embarrassed by my own noises — the zipper to my tent, the crunch of the leaves under my flip flops — my flip flops slapping against my heels. At some point — yes, after the bathroom I remembered to take off my shoes. Remembered even on the painful rocks of Death Valley (now ten years ago) I had learned that the ground was safe — harmless, painless, if you step softly and at the pace it wants you to go. Each surface having its own "speed limit"... I stopped often to hear the many birds, insects, and silences in between. And stopped to finally see the trees — on my own terms rather than by instruction. They were standing in the morning sunlight, and I suddenly realized how they could be recognized as "people" — they are so clearly people, and I felt their presence, their invitation for me to trust them — just trust that they are truthfully there. And that they have no intent of harming me — they are just simply there... And I stood seeing them and hearing the birds surrounding me. One pulled my attention ahead of me — not frequent but loud — a hawk? An owl? — Something so strong and sharp but unknown to me. So, I approached at the speed of silence on the dirt path that crosses the meadow, looking up to the treetops to see who was making this sound. But as I moved slowly and embedded in the experience, I saw ahead, across the meadow, a fox. A small fox. And then I felt it must be the fox's call I'd heard. I stopped and waited and watched and sure enough I saw the fox call out. The rest of my walk was peaceful — curious — letting the sights and sounds and feeling beneath my feet talk to me... I know one absolute truth — you don't need books to learn to be in the woods. I found a heart rock on the trail and left it there. It is an old, worn-out symbol of something past — an old way — that at the time was good, but no longer holds meaning. Or the meaning that it held is no longer useful. I joked with Sven before I left that I was only looking for liver shaped rocks from now on. But I left the rock behind on that path, "I see you," I said, and continued walking. The yellow straw was extremely soft under my feet. I wondered if I could find my way in the dark simply by this feeling.

Ben:
On day two, we take the trainees out on a second walk. And again, it's kind of like Sunshine and Rainbows. But then in the afternoon, we get into the Way of the Guide content session. I think of that shift as like when you step into the ocean; it kind of slowly, slowly declines and then at some point, it drops off and

just gets so deep, so fast. So, I think of that second half of that day, where we discuss the way of the guide, as kind of like that moment where the ocean floor drops. And suddenly, people come into a very immediate reality or understanding that this is so much more complicated than it looks on the outside. I think during the way of the guide piece most people come to realize that the art of facilitation is not about skills as much as it is about the guide's attitude. This attitude is characterized by trust, patience, and a genuine focus on process over end results.

That's the turning point that I don't think there's any way to prepare people for — that moment that the floor drops — the way of the guide is so shocking to people because it's so countercultural. This is the moment in the training when people realize that everything that they've been taught about how to lead, how to be in a leadership position, is working against what they're going to be doing here because this leadership model is not about control whatsoever. So, then the rest of the week takes on a certain element of de-schooling or deconditioning, or re-wilding. There are many, many, many layers of stripping away people's perceptual biases around how to work with a group and how to lead. Whereas most people have been conditioned to think that a leader is responsible for making something particular happen, in this model, a leader is someone who creates a space where anything is possible, and everything is accepted. And that is where the real magic is cultivated.

8:53 p.m. — Journal Entry: Second Night
Looking forward to sleeping tonight. It was a very full day — walking with the group this morning was calming. The theme for me became "taking care of myself." It was a day with me and with the Earth's medicine. Embodying the notion of kincentric — and the idea that we need to connect to be in relation with the more-than-human world to actually be in right relationship. That we affect each other and should in fact touch and move and bond with each other. I saw it when Ben

picked a dandelion and blew the seeds to the wind. I saw it when I picked up a feather and let it fall, watched it land again from my hand. So much learning — too much to remember and hoping that it stays in my body/mind. I know I will need many, many more of these experiences to make it real — to make it true from inside of me to outside of me.

I am intrigued by the ritual of a Vision Fast to deeply connect with the land. It is clear to me that this is a passion of mine, and my freedom is paramount to most everything else now. The freedom to move, to learn, to grow, to follow my spirit and not let anything block me now. This is much more than a career choice. This is a way of being that I've longed for — and made a great sacrifice for. To not embody it would be to dishonor everyone who agreed with me in taking these risks. A dishonor to Marley and to my mother. A dishonor to all the women who came before me and who will come after me.

I am slowly meeting the people here — slowly making them into no longer strangers. Although I don't know if any will be friends — I am touching antennae and liking the process. They are good people. Different people, but good people. I like Elizabeth. I would like to know more about Nicole. And Ben is an amazing guide — an amazing soul — I am happily surprised. I hope he will continue to teach me in Los Angeles. I don't know how else I will proceed. I am trusting the process, trusting the program, and trusting the trees.

Amos came into camp tonight. He is a visionary and has the brain to put it into coherent language, science, fact, accessible to every kind of mind. Some of his stories scared me. But I'm okay with that honestly. I'm sure I sound "crazy" when I speak from my heart & soul. He and I know the same truth though we arrived on different paths. We meet at the nexus and I am grateful for his mind and his brain.

I'd like to know Nicole — her path, her vision, but above all I'd like to know my own. Retain and remember my own voice — remember I don't need to follow anyone but me from this day forward. I follow only my own soul — my own wisdom. Take my own journey. That is my right and my responsibility. And I am grateful for this conviction.

I feel happy and healthy and, as they say, in a perpetual liminal space as I have stepped outside my ordinary world for this week. I am at my edge and appreciating the learning — the embodied experience of "don't know mind"— even the shower was completely new. I had the experience of three minutes being an eternity. Twenty-five cents/ minute for water — it probably only took two minutes — it is all new — all strange — all possibility. Beginner's mind, and as everyone winds down outside my tent — talking and sharing — I miss Marley. She's my home base now and I also feel tremendous gratitude for my friends who spurred me on to take this journey. ♡

6:58 a.m. — Journal Entry: Second Morning
It is cold. I kept the tarp off the tent so that it wouldn't be as hot and so that I could wake up to the sky and trees. And it is cold. I slept. But not as well, mainly because I had already formed an expectation of "sleeping well" from the night before. Truthfully, I probably slept much the same. The cold and the bit of familiarity I feel for the campgrounds made me rush this morning. I know the people now — although I don't know them at all — and I feel myself rushing to join them — even though they aren't up. I know they will be soon. I am trying to recreate the feeling of yesterday morning. But this morning is cold — or I am cold in it — and it's harder for me to meander in the cold. Especially barefoot and needing to use the bathroom — my beautiful bladder holding firm for me again through the night and letting me sleep. I found the trail in the meadow, but it was colder to the touch than last night. The bathroom — now my "favorite" bathroom — was warm and peaceful although someone — a child I hope — put a paper towel in the toilet. My impulse was to fish it out with a stick, but I thought it better to let the park managers handle it.
I almost forgot to see the trees this time when I stepped out of the bathroom, a little warmer, and about to head back to my tent. But thankfully I looked up. Stopped. Saw them again in the morning sunshine. Said "hello," "good morning" of sorts before I stepped back onto the path. No fox, but a small flock of little birds accompanied ...

or should I say shared the trail with me this time. They flitted here and there I suppose looking for food? While I slowly walked behind them. I thought about Amos again — his strange and compelling stories — questioning his sanity and, seeing that place doubt about my own. Is this crazy? Remembering to stay with my truth — to ward off thinking I should be like anyone else. Watching how fear operates. Remembering that fear complicates things unnecessarily. It's enough for me to notice what I see in the more-than-human world — they are my mentors, guides, and therapists — they have no "hidden agenda." They are ego-less and therefore safe. At least that is a question I have. Are they ego-less? How would I know? The familiar woven into the unfamiliar makes me think and doubt and think again...

Ben:

It all comes back to one of my favorite expressions: "You can't open a rose with a crowbar." This is, again, about ego and control. Most people want something to happen; they want those who they guide to receive healing or transformation or reconciliation or whatever it is, but these are all projections of the guide. It is fully possible for a guide to manipulate people into having powerful experiences, but the attitude of the guide is about trusting that organic, authentic experiences are always superior to those that are coerced, even in the most subtle ways. This is a moment where there's a lot of cognitive dissonance for the trainees because they must learn to abandon their own hopes so that they can create space for the reality of authentic experiences.

What I've noticed is that a lot of people come to the work of forest therapy imagining they're going to embody a sort of a healer archetype. They come thinking, "I'm going to be doing this special, wonderful, magical thing," which indicates to me that they often begin their journey from a place of ego, of believing that it is their facilitation alone that creates the essential magic of what people experience. In the practice, however, guides learn to de-center themselves from the process of the participant so that it is within the relationship between nature and participant that the essential magic is found. For many guides, this takes years and many walks to truly understand. Oftentimes, guides begin with a great deal of doubt and mistrust, of themselves, their participants and of nature itself. This invariably leads people to subtly manipulate the experience of their participants until they begin to embrace the radical simplicity and unconditional trust of the practice. When guides really understand that they are not responsible for creating any particular outcome and they become comfortable with the wide range of authentic experiences that can arise, that is when they begin to really walk the path.

So that day, day three, is kind of where the ocean really opens up. And then people are, I think, from that point on, really kind of like swimming in the deep. When you can't see the shore anymore. It's very disorienting, and in some ways, it's a little bit terrifying. I think at that point, people are expending a lot of energy just to stay afloat, and they were not anticipating this. But in other ways, this is where a lot of the personal inner work starts happening. This is where there's a shift from "I really need to use this week to be focused on the acquisition of skills" to, "I need to really start unpacking myself, and understanding how I've been tamed and understanding how to let go of some of that taming so that I can actually work with people and support the Forest in being the therapist."

8:58 p.m. — Journal Entry: Third Night
Sometimes I am feeling cranky — like I've had enough of this way of living — the stress of the unfamiliar, although there's nothing about the familiar I really want to return to. Went on a store run and didn't like that either — no real desire to connect with the "ordinary world" — yet being with these strangers outside all the time — strange

food, strange cooking is ... well ... I don't know what it is. Just perpetually different. As Marley said, "Like summer camp" to which I replied, "That I never went to. For a reason." The concepts are inspiring. I'd love to sit and talk for hours and hours about the philosophies that underpin the core activities and exercises — or invitations — the concept of guiding the person to discovering their own "medicine' through authentic contact & connection with the more-than-human world. Priceless — really stepping far outside the role of "healer" and into witness, and invitation maker. It is Zen in action. A wonderful skill to learn and reminds me of the old homeschooling methods I used with Marley when she was little. Fostering curiosity and questions rather than pushing for some answer. I am looking forward to tomorrow.

6:45 a.m. — Journal Entry: Third Morning

My bladder had had enough and woke me at 4:30 — I couldn't deny it any longer and thought, "Okay. So, I will see this place in the dark." I didn't like it. The crunch of the leaves under my weight was too loud. The pathway, much too dark. In consideration of my fellow campers, I used the red flashlight and so could hardly see much more than with no light. But I used the toilet and that felt good.

I walked back now fully awake by the cold night air and the stress of finding my way. The pillow and blanket were icy. The only relief was to put the covers over my head and heat myself with my own breath. The creek beside me was comforting. I may have dozed a bit but mostly waited for daylight and as it appeared I surrendered to wakefulness and went out again — now befriended by the sun to take the longer walk to my favorite bathroom across the meadow. Just as cold, but now visible — and audible — as the crows have awakened as well and they circle above and call to each other.

I still feel this undefinable feeling of unease. Can't quite place it — maybe just missing some effect of creature comfort that is usually with me but now missing. Maybe missing the accumulated effect of always being warm and entertained and peopled with my familiar voices and actions. Probably even actions I am bothered with at home — the car, the drive, the coffee run, the walk to work — I don't know. Or maybe simply a warm bed and hot shower every day and food I'm used to eating. Yes. As I write it, I recognize it. I am missing warmth, cleanliness, and familiar food. Cooking. I miss cooking. And still, I appreciate being here — the bay canopy — the fragrance never fails me — it is one of my new friends. I will have to consider how to repay it. I am not looking forward to my camp breakfast forage. It will be bananas & toasted pita as always. Why bother to eat? This morning's walk will be co-led by each other — I will lead "What's in motion" — trying to stay with the simplicity of it — Fear Complicates Things Unnecessarily.

Ben:

Day four, we send people to guide each other for the first time. And you know, it's this strange moment where you're doing something for the first time, and you have to come face-to-face with all the insecurities of doing something new for the first time. A lot of people struggle with this, either because they are attached to "being good at it" or "doing it right" or because they are experiencing echoes of the educational trauma of their pasts. Of course, there is also a lot of joy and excitement at this moment, because it is at this moment that the trainees become their own teachers and begin experimenting and playing and seeing for themselves what's possible.

When we debrief these walks, we try to draw attention particularly to what felt right, what filled guides with a sense of easeful relaxation, as these are the experiences in which they often experience the forest as the therapist and have felt a de-centering of their own role in the process. It is an interesting experience, of course, because everyone on the walk is a guide in training, and so they are wearing two hats simultaneously: they are both guide and participant, they are both experiencing and analyzing the experience.

9:29 p.m. — Journal Entry: Fourth Night

I am dirty and tired of sleeping in the woods. Mainly because I'm tired of being so cold in the middle of the night. It was too late and dark to put my tarp over the tent. So, I have to face another night of freezing. So, okay. I am also tired of being with people who have a way of being comfortable with each other that I don't have. I enjoy them. Truly. But I don't get them. Or maybe I just don't have a similar past. They are brave, and outdoor people — they run and climb and deep-sea dive and fish for piranha and travel to Iceland. They do road trips cross country and run into bears and elks and deer and the list goes on. They sing for each other and tell stories. They are that drama class I hid from as a kid. But they don't hide. And so, okay. But they also meditate and walk with Thich Nhat Hanh and want to guide people back into the woods like me. So, okay. I don't know who I really am — and honestly, I don't care. I just want to follow this path and see where it leads. I don't care if I am a misfit — I don't care if I'm not. I don't want to stay in my safety zone — because frankly it's not safe. And I don't want to leave my safety zone because honestly that's not the right road either. I will just follow my heart — stay close to my soul and see where I go....

7:53 a.m. — Journal Entry: Fourth Morning

I had an epiphany today about living each day like a forest walk — using the standard sequence: Hospitality, Introduction, Pleasures of Presence, What's in Motion, It Depends, and Tea Ceremony to end the day — what will make this feel complete? My emotions ran strong around the idea of offering hospitality to myself each day "I'm glad you're here." On the way back from my morning bathroom, I came back to the campsite to find Michael, Sarah and Michelle already talking and having tea — it was nice to have them there and open more conversation about life, the practice and what each of us is discovering and questioning separately and together — to share minds — in an open, friendly way. Guy joined and he added some nice ideas as well. We are all so different — yet strung together by a thread of mindful awareness — which leads, I believe, to the woods. I am glad to be feeling some connection beginning. Some familiarity that can lead to openness and trust. What will today bring?

Ben:

Then day five, they go on one more trainer-led walk. At this point, the trainees are typically at the point where they're becoming very, very attentive, and critical about what's going on. In other words, they have become masterful at wearing the two hats at once. And because they have become more aware that forest therapy needs not to be performed, it's not all Sunshine and Rainbows anymore. On this walk, we often see a greater depth of vulnerability, as trainees are embodying a greater sort of permission towards themselves. It's also at this point that they begin seeing the diversity of technique and style that each trainer is demonstrating while still remaining within the practice. This gives trainees a more nuanced question than what they might have entered with. Whereas in the beginning, they were thinking of how they might imitate the trainers in order to "do it right," they begin to ask themselves, "how will I guide?" This question invites them into a deeper relationship with themselves and with the more-than-human world, as they begin to see nature as an active partner and not a passive subject.

9:36 p.m. — Journal Entry: Fifth Night

A long but beautiful day in the heat. Quarry Hill — it is kind of enchanting. Nice to experience a "forest walk" in the garden and it was so peaceful. But the heat has given me a headache and the headache makes me cranky. I have a kind of sense of futility coming over me. Feel very far away from what I'd originally thought this practice would be — it is highly structured — in some very important ways — but it has its own language and philosophy, more akin to homeschooling than I'd imagined. My thoughts were about mindfulness in nature — but although one would be mindful, it is not that. It is truly teaching people to connect with the more-than-human world. The invitation is designed to help someone find their relationship with the forest — much more about that partnership than just about the human. I am starting to get the idea. Guy asked me what I plan to do with this — I think it's something we're all thinking about. But my answer remains the same — I will bring it home and start to practice with it — I will let the practice itself tell me what it wants me to do with it. And if it never develops into anything big — that's okay, it will be what it will be. It's something to get comfortable with — for me to make a home in the woods & share what I discover. First things First.

7:40 a.m. — Journal Entry: Fifth Morning

I feel sad. I don't know why. Maybe having a brush with the "outside world" made me too aware of my struggles at home in my relationship. My feelings of being shamed, misperceived & unfairly treated. I heard a family in conflict this morning as I walked back to the campsite from the bathroom. It made me reflect on how and why people fight — what is it that's going wrong? What does it point to ultimately? What is it that we need? One thought I had was simply to be understood and hear a heartfelt recognition of the transgression and a truthful regret — "I'm sorry." It makes me think of Thich Nhat Hanh's words, "Tell me darling, how have I hurt you?" The openness and willingness to hear that, to receive it as true and to express a truthful regret at having caused it. But that, although extremely true, is only one thought. Wondering if there's some other benefit of conflict — discord — bumping into each other on some level — like gentle wrestling — to build something? To strengthen identity? To find one's own voice/one's own medicine? But enough about humans. Although they are encroaching closer and closer. I didn't sleep well — too hard — don't remember dreams — I woke later than usual. I didn't want to get up. And the thought of simply not opening my tent today crossed my mind. I listened to the sound of a heavy bird flying low over my tent. The rustle of feathers in flight. Possibly my favorite sound. I wondered if Rocket would know the word for that sound and then immediately wanted not to know it. The sound is enough. I don't have to name it. The other birds continue to call near and far — their rhythmic sounds that are so much a part of being here. They are comforting and reassuring guardians — no matter what I feel or think or fear or fill in the blank — I hear them, familiar, and it lets me know everything is okay. And so am I.

10:06 p.m. — Journal Entry: Sixth Night
What a wonderful evening. Michelle led Shabbat — it was beautiful. I feel blessed and happy. I felt useful and blessed to be of service to her to make sure she could observe her holiday. And it was truly lovely and shared by everyone — today was a good day. Had "Invitation Clinic" which was crafting a series of invitations one after another — a beautiful way to spend the morning. And a good way to learn. Tomorrow we will lead a walk for "the public" — I have no idea who or how many that will be. It seems I should be nervous, but I'm not and hoping to keep it that way. I trust the process, the forest, the experience, and the curriculum. I also trust my group — it's amazing how these bonds form in only a day or two more. I feel much closer to almost everyone. So tomorrow I will lead Pleasures of Presence and am very much looking forward to guiding people to open their senses in an easy gentle way. I am also very much looking forward to more training. Council of the Trees and Water seems so appealing. And I'm thinking I will walk with Ben for the rest of the year to have more experiences with him. For myself I am thinking of offering a series of classes — I think it's the best way to really introduce people to the woods. One walk is not enough. I see how much is gained by doing more than one experience.

6:58 a.m. — Journal Entry: Sixth Morning
Had a bad night's sleep — the mattress didn't seem to hold air for as long as usual and I found myself sleeping hipbone to earth for

much of the time. I will be glad to sleep in a bed — although I have not done my usual tossing and turning — and haven't felt the usual anxiety, worry, or tenseness since I've been here. The nights and days are extremely peaceful — especially inside myself — unless, or until, I think of home, work, my relationship ... anything from "back there in the real world" makes me tense inside and feel some of that old familiar angst. Angst is the perfect word. Don't know why I haven't thought of it until now. Today — the public walk — is connecting me to my public self — and I don't like it. I see what a huge divide there is between my public self and my forest self — I hope that changes. I hope as I go deeper into the woods I will find myself and having found myself and spent enough time, won't lose myself so easily when faced with a public, or professional task. I don't want to be dis-integrated anymore. It is much too painful. But here I am — and reminded of the domestication I feel. How do I look? What will I say? How am I going to be judged? I don't like it. And though I may have felt something like that meeting these people, I gave myself a different premise. Kind of "anything is okay" or "I don't care if I'm liked or not..." whatever that whole trip is that causes me so much pain. Plus, there is always an escape into nature whenever I need — the trees, the fields, the more-than-human beings that are my priority to connect with. At any given moment, I can wander off and sit with a rock, bird, patch of grass or whatever called to me, and I can do it without shame or explanation to the people around me. That is the true medicine.

Ben:

And then day six is when we do the content on Circle what we now refer to as Gathering Circle. The way I think of it, is a practice that embodies the ethical framework of Way of the Guide. Circle is about unconditional acceptance of what others are experiencing and the validation of all experiences as equally meaningful. Circle is how guides express to their participants that there is no pressure to have any particular outcome or experience. It relies on the guide authentically embracing whatever is coming up for people, whether it's grief or childlike frivolity or anything at all.

Whenever participants can sense that the guide has an expectation, they are prone to performing whatever they think the guide wants. The way people relate to leaders, they are conditioned to look to the leader to validate their experiences. This conditioning is so deep that people rarely even notice themselves doing it. By offering everyone a chance to express themselves, even if it is in silence, Circle provides an opportunity for each story to be heard. And the art of facilitating this kind of Circle is not as simple as passing around a sharing piece; the real art is in welcoming every story with equal dignity and respect.

This is hard for people at first, because of an ego trap. What happens is that when someone shares something deep or emotional, the guide tends to get excited because they think to themselves, "This is working! Someone is having a powerful experience!" And then they react, verbally or physically, in a way that suggests they value that story. It can be as subtle as people nodding their heads when they are listening. But what happens when the next person shares something and there is no head nodding?

Facilitating Circle is challenging for new guides because they have to learn to value all stories, even when they don't understand them or don't perceive them as being particularly powerful. The truth is the guide has no idea. There have been so many times in my own guiding practice where the people having the deepest experience say absolutely nothing at all.

And the content session on Circle is usually interesting because it challenges a taming we have about listening. Most people think the point of listening is to figure out what to say in response, so that you might be helpful in some way. But in Circle, the point of listening is just to listen, to give space to another person to say what they want to say, without any interference or manipulation at all.

And it's hard because people are not accustomed to bearing witness in this way. I was just talking to a friend yesterday about this; she's a breathwork teacher, and she was describing how she has a hard time really being compassionate for people when they're sharing their stories because she feels like she's getting entangled in the stories and then she's processing the story of someone else.

For me, the thing that's really countercultural about holding space is that you have to decouple empathy and compassion. Because if I'm receiving your story with a sense of empathy, I'm entangled in it. And when I get entangled, then I'm in the story. I have an agenda because of who I am and because of my own story. If I'm entangled in your story, I might want to resolve it, and now I'm influencing the field and I'm influencing the emergence of the story.

So, when we teach Circle... and I've been on a long journey with this, sometimes people just hate me for it... They're like, "You're a monster! You're telling me not to comfort people? Not to fix their problem? Not to react with compassion?" ... and I say, "Perhaps the most compassionate thing you can do is simply listen. Perhaps in bearing witness to someone's story, without criticism or validation, you allow them to become their most authentic selves."

11:55 p.m. — Journal Entry: Seventh Night
So hard to let this day end since it's the last night we'll all be together. We had a wonderful day in the woods with each other and the trees — then lots of down time together to talk and share our hopes and dreams for this walk and our place in the world. A nice dinner out, a walk up to the observatory to see Jupiter and Saturn through the big lenses and finally a nice fire with Nicole playing for us. Singing together. Yes, it is the overnight camp experience

I never had only one thousand times better since I am old, and confident and have no fear. Yes, I said that. By now I feel so secure and comfortable. I don't feel any fear. I am hoping to take this home with me. Not sure what will actually happen next, but again I am hopeful it will be strong. So, blowing up this air mattress for the last time — and tucking down in my cozy little "home." I will miss it. I will miss it. And I will miss all these quirky people. Twenty-two dear & strong personalities. Would be so cool if we all lived close and cared to stay together. But who knows. I am hopeful to stay connected to these people — some if not all. What a surprising and needed experience.

8:27 a.m. — Journal Entry: Seventh Morning

I am balancing between staying present with these last few hours and anticipating leaving. All that awaits at home. I notice an immediate shift in my body, anxiety, tension, worry, unhappiness. It is informative and makes me sad. I hope that I can bring more of what I've felt this last week home with me. And using my sense of self, sense of place, body radar to be better at honoring "yes" and "no." I am looking forward to our last experience — a medicine walk — three hours alone with the more-than-humans. I took a little forest walk this morning to begin and chose (as they invited us to do) to fast through this. It should be easy. I am somewhat aware of the potential for rattlesnake encounters, but probably won't meet one on this journey. I am open to what the forest will provide...

Ben:

On the last day, there's the Solo Walk. I think for a lot of people, it's the most powerful part of the whole week. I think part of it is because people are exhausted and so they have no trouble surrendering to the moment. They've spent a whole week learning something that really challenges a lot of their cultural conditioning and then they are craving emptiness. In this state, three hours of solitude within a container of absolute freedom, is something that tends to open pieces of the experience that have been closed until this point. It's usually on that experience where you see people start to ... even people who are very academic in their approach ... that's where mystical things happen.

I think for a lot of people, the experience of that walk is, well, that's where an incredible amount of the value of the experience lies, because it kind of illuminates this intense simplicity. I always tell people with the Solo Walk, "Don't have any expectations about this. Just go out there and just be there. You know, just be there; so simple. Just go on a walk for three hours. Don't talk. Don't go inside. Don't eat. Just go." Right? And the stories that come back are really, I mean, I think this is where like, if you didn't take the training and people were telling you those stories, it would prompt people to be a little incredulous about it. Like, "Come on ... that didn't really happen." You know, the stories that come back from the Solo Walk are just oftentimes ... just intensely poetic and powerful. People don't really expect it to be like that.

I think part of it is that people have such a bias around the power of simplicity. People are coming to the training and they're thinking, "Well, I've been outside before ... I've gone on a walk by myself in the woods before ... how different can this be?" But then the container and the construction of the threshold that they cross from ordinary to liminal worlds ... just that very, very simple process radically changes everything about the way they perceive their time. And even people that live outside, spend all their time outside... This can be huge. It's life changing for a lot of people. I know a lot of guides who still talk about those three hours of their lives.

After the Solo Walk, we hold our final circle and say our goodbyes. I think for some people, this is an abrupt transition, and something I think we manage better in the new model of our training. But regardless, the transition from Solo Walk to a threshold of incorporation is powerful. It's kind of like ... if we take that metaphor of the ocean again, as if we are at the greatest depth and then, at the end of the week, you hit this Whirlpool, and then it just rockets you out of the ocean and spits you out on the beach of some other continent and you're just like, "what just happened?" I think of it like an initiation; there is a sort of climax that ushers you in to the next phase of the experience, where you go home and just when you thought the experience couldn't get any deeper, you start learning to be in deep relationship with the land you actually live on, with the beings you actually spend your life with.

Our last invitation was this solo "medicine walk" for three hours in whatever part of the forest called to us. We were invited to fast for the walk bringing only drinking water, our day pack, a timepiece, and our journal with us. Nothing more. This would be time spent with the more-than-human world completely on our own. For the training, the solo walk is a shortened experience of a traditional fasting medicine walk which starts at sunrise and concludes at sunset. This walk is done at the end of the six-month practicum. The day-long is also a shorter version of a traditional Vision Fast which is four days and nights in the wild without food or shelter. Many guides are drawn to do a Vision Fast at some point, but it isn't part of this curriculum.

There is something about going without food and shelter into nature that creates a perceptual context for receiving the experience differently. Even though this would only be half the day, it added a felt sense of "time outside of the ordinary," or specialness to the experience.

We gathered among the trees at 9 a.m. A wide circle of branches had been laid out on the ground. At the center of the circle was a round, colorful cloth and on it a tray of small scrolls. Three scrolls were bundled together by a piece of green yarn (I still have my yarn on my bedside table to remind me). There was one set for each of us. The bundles had a tag with our names written on it, and each of the scrolls had a message or prompt written inside for us. We were instructed to open one scroll at a time when we felt called to do so during our walk. We were also told to keep an eye on the time and that we needed to return to this same circle exactly three hours later or a search party would have to be sent out. "Stay found," we were warned. Meaning wander anywhere you like but know where you are so that you don't risk getting lost and making us have to go find you!

The circle was described as the threshold between our camp and the liminal world. Once we stepped into the circle, we would become "invisible" to each other, so that even if we ran across someone in the woods, we "couldn't see them." We were told to step into the circle when we felt drawn to do so, find our scrolls, and then cross out of the circle (now invisible) to begin our medicine walk.

There was something so transformative about that suggestion. It felt ceremonial, exciting, and limitless. I watched as a few people began crossing into and out of the circle. I felt myself wanting to cross, felt my energy building, but just before I did, I caught a glimpse of what looked like a long winding gray snake. A fallen tree branch. And although I knew it was a branch, something about it felt important. Wise. Alive. I felt the urge to pick it up, but for a moment I judged myself. Questioned my impulse. Was that allowed? Do I really need it? Shouldn't I just follow the instructions? But, committed to listening to myself, I walked over to where it lay, picked it up and crossed swiftly into the circle with it.

Inside the circle I approached the pile of scrolls, found the bundle of three with my name on it, took a deep breath, and stepped outside the circle again invisible. Without the burden of being "seen" by anyone, my mind unfolded into a realm of complete non-judgement and curiosity for what lay ahead for the next three hours.

Final Journal Entry: Medicine Walk

Snake medicine ... carried with me in a tree branch. "I want to go with you, Sweetness. Take me with you. We will walk together," tree-snake said. Off the path and into the untouched field. I become a hawk flying fast over land, surveying, watching, protecting, enjoying... Then become a giant human with steps too heavy — lightening them, I become a spirit and move easily and gently onward — Peaceful calm. Crossing out of the human realm I walk — Lizard stops me. We sit together — Lizard scratches and moves on bringing me to four trees: Bay, Pine, Fern, and Holly? Closeness, intimacy, uniqueness, oneness — Flies tell me it is time to go...

Deeper into the woods it cools. Listening. Waiting. The woods speak of patience and stillness. Blue dragonfly appears — speaking of movement and stillness. Moving to a rock, lands, opens wings two times or three or six or five ... then still — motionless — until three shades of blue and then off down the path to sit with rocks and wood and leaves beyond — telling me it's time to go...

Mud said, "Feel me — hold me in your hands and give me a face so that I can see the forest the way you do." Feather, green and acorn headdress, she wants to be in the tree. She is happy with her new green moss body — offering her a blackberry, she brings me to sit still with her and the tree. Festival. Dancing. High into the air. Blue birds tell me it is time to move ... down the stream... Water-rock has a lot to say — skimmer bugs gliding around and listen closely to the water. Bubbles. Churning. Making air pockets. No hand. No faucet. Water moves of its own free will. Still, moving quickly, becomes still again.

The first scroll's message was about commitment. And so, I made a promise to the woods and water and all beings around me that I wouldn't leave them anymore — that I would spend time no matter what, every day in true connection. And in return I asked them to let me know when I can leave the city.

The hill sloped up in the sun and it was challenging. It's okay — go slowly. Listen to your heart, take care of your body. Water tank & pipes — I feel conflict and harmony and conflict. But behind the tank all is quiet and still. The next scroll's message I had already done instinctively with the last "what would I like to ask from the land" — so the only part is what I can offer in return... I am asking for the land to tell me what it would like ... deep listening... Fly says it's time to move, the answer is down the path...

Integrity. Flexibility. Forgiveness. Communication. Rustling being shows me nine Bay trees— young trees — food — foraging — Baby tree grove — the nursery of young ones — interbeing. Rustling bird finally appears and red bird tells me it's time to go...

Truth has been easy at times — many times — and challenging other times due to forgetting to speak from my heart — rather forgetting to listen to my heart before speaking — and sometimes a challenge for fear of being judged. For fear that my Truth separates me from others rather than bonds me. Making peace with the truth of times to be separate — separately — me — distinguishing myself — getting closer to the truth of complete interconnectedness. Meaning finding the truth of interconnectedness in my body. Remembering the more-than-human world. Keeping that connection, strengthening that bond in my body. Strengthening my bonds with the few people my body — my _whole_ body says "yes" to. And keeping light touch connections/bonds with those who aren't _whole_ body — and connecting from a distance with people who are a "no" — learning not to override these signals. That is a truthful path with humans.

Strengthening my bond with more-than-humans but being wise that no means no with them as well. This is my distinction. This will be my honest path — my true path. This will be a way to live peacefully. But right now, it is still a learning. And there is no hurry.

No rush ... diligence, commitment, patience, and reminders will help me deepen my truth telling inside and outside of my body...

Bird above knocks three times on the branches of the tree beside me. Making a melody here and there like a tapping drum — woodpecker — time to simply listen...

The crossings back and forth through the threshold we made between liminal space and ordinary space are quite emotional. Coming back out of the walk, I felt a bit of something — not exactly sure what the feeling is — maybe gratitude, recognition? — I don't know. And a feeling of not wanting to re-enter the ordinary world. Want to stay silent — doesn't really matter — just an observation.

The Medicine Walk, or Solo Walk, was indeed transformational. Personally, I liked the way my cohort was trained even though we were metaphorically spit out of a whirlpool onto another continent. There was something poetic about it. And for me, it perpetuated this sense of absolute beginner's mind.

My sense of being a hawk flying over the land was exhilarating. The tiny plants at my feet appeared as large trees and fields below me and I seemed to see through Hawk eyes. Then the perception shifted, and I saw myself towering over the trees, a giant with the snake-stick by my side. I recognized how heavy my weight was on the plants below me and lightened my steps. Intentional softness, my perception shifted again, and I felt as if I were a spirit, a ghost able to pass through without harm.

As I walked deeper into the woods, my attention felt drawn to movement and stillness. I used the animals' movements to signal my own, find the next place that held something for me to sit with, stay motionless observing, communing, until another being gave me the cue to move on.

I allowed myself not to know what I was doing. Allowed the bit of uncomfortableness and unfamiliarity to be okay. Again, being invisible I allowed myself permission to be and do whatever came to me without judgment or propriety interfering. At times I found myself crying deeply to the trees, listening to the mud, or studying the wing rhythms of damselflies like some kind of Morse code. Things that made no sense. I followed Mary Oliver's advice and simply let the soft animal of my body do what it loved.

Three hours later most of us were crossing back through the "portal" and regaining our visibility met with a hearty "Hello! Nice to see you again!" from our trainers. It was playful, silly, and completely essential to create the container we needed.

After all of us had crossed back through the circle threshold, and regained our visibility, we met for our final session. As we sat together under the bay laurel trees for the last time, now a cohesive bonded group with each other and the land, we shared what was in our hearts. I felt how completely relaxed my body and mind were. I had noticed it for the past two days. The level of calm was unfamiliar. Though I consider myself a calm person, as do others, this feeling was different. There was no tension anywhere to be found. I felt warm, heavy, and supple. My smile came easily, my heart was open and soft. I imagined this must have been the way I felt as a child before the world had shaped me into my domesticated self. It reassured me that my own internal wilderness was safe, loving, and full. I hoped to bring this feeling home to share.

As the talking piece came around the circle to me, I shared my surprise at the level of emotional safety I felt during the solo walk. I told my cohort how I cried deeply to the trees about what it was like to live in a city, how unimaginable they would find all the concrete and noise. How hard it was to bear every day. Things I didn't truly know I felt until it all came pouring out in the safety of being visible only to the natural world. The unconditional acceptance of the water, mud, trees, plants, and animals allowed an uncensored outpour. I recommitted to a daily practice for myself and to letting the practice guide me in how I might bring it to others.

As I tore down my tent and loaded up my car, I felt the mixture of sadness and gratitude that accompanies any transformational experience. I hoped I would stay in touch with my cohort — and at least we would have monthly group calls to reconnect us. But everyone was spreading out again, returning to their homes in different states and different countries. I felt very lucky to have Ben in Los Angeles and one other guide, Jackie. They became my seed pod.

What follows the week-long immersion is a six-month mentored practicum with a detailed and rigorous curriculum and lots and lots of unstructured time alone with nature. I felt grateful to have the practicum ahead of me for support. It gave me another kind of scaffolding to lean into and trust.

The next six months were the perfect balance of confusion and containment. Ben became my mentor and continued to hold that space of true compassion, never letting himself or his ideas contaminate my growing relationship with the rest of nature.

Oftentimes I was frustrated and felt lost, wishing he would train me the way the rest of my past teachers and supervisors had. But thankfully he didn't. He let me find my own rhythm in the natural world and supported me unconditionally. No matter what I said or did, he made open suggestions that forced me to turn to myself and the rest of nature for whatever answers might come ... and enabled me to be comfortable when no answer appeared. What he referred to as "living the question." I highly recommend this as a way of life. It is counterculture, almost heretical, to a society that over-values expertise, superiority, and hierarchy. Living the question revives and refreshes a way of being in the world that is comfortable, at ease, playful, and always growing. I might even venture to say it is the only way to real resiliency and acceptance of self, others, and circumstances. Over the years my continued practice of forest therapy and guiding others has deepened my understanding of how to cultivate an unconditional love of life itself.

Reflection Invitation

What would you be like if you felt unconditional love of life itself? Would anything change in your mind? In your relationships?

7

The I-Thou Relationship: I See the Trees and the Trees See Me

Imagine Trees standing together in a forest. They don't talk, but they feel each other's presence. When you look at them, you might say they aren't doing anything. But they are growing and providing clean air for living things to breathe.

Thich Nhat Hanh, Vietnamese Buddhist monk,
author, poet, and peace activist

Martin Buber was an Austrian, Jewish, and Israeli philosopher who wrote his most famous essay in 1923 — *Ich und Du* (I-Thou). This essay centered on two ways of approaching existence: the "I-It" relationship where one sees the other as an object to be used or experienced and the "I-Thou" relationship in which the other is seen as a mutual partnership between beings.

An "I-Thou" attitude describes a world that doesn't objectify an "It" but acknowledges a living relationship between two entities. It's essential to recognize that Buber's view is not limited to partnerships between people, and very much includes relationships with trees, the sky, a river, and so on. This is a world of relations. This is a world of attachment. Relationship with another is paramount and according to Buber is where meaning is found.

The cultivation of this way of being with the more-than-human world is essential to the work of repairing our relationship with the rest of nature. Likewise, the guide's de-programming from any "I-It" bias with the rest of nature is central to being able to effectively guide others toward healing their own "I-It" tendencies that our culture teaches. For example, using Nature to feel better (I-It) versus spending time in connection with non-human beings and discovering what may serve the reciprocal needs of each other (I-Thou).

The six months practicum that follows the week-long intensive provides the time, space and container for this "I-Thou" perspective (among other skills) to develop and deepen. I'd like to share a bit about the practicum. Although there is too much to tell everything, there are some important aspects that I believe are relevant at this point especially in terms of the personal growth the curriculum cultivates and how it fosters an "I-Thou" relationship with the more-than-human beings, without anthropomorphizing them.

Attributing human characteristics or behaviors to more-than-human beings may be a doorway into connecting with the rest of nature. So, I don't want to discourage it if that's what opens the relationship for you or for anyone you're guiding. However, over time and with more experiences there is a way to encounter and relate to other species as *they* are: non-human and having something uniquely their own to offer. I would venture to say that these two ways of connecting intertwine and come and go throughout the relationship. Just as we may notice how sometimes we see our dog as a dog and sometimes we see her as a furry human. It's all okay. With time, in connection with other beings, we can come to see their unique intelligence not as inferior to humans, but as equally valuable and oftentimes wiser. And we can begin to see what we can genuinely give to them in return. It's important to remember that reciprocity is key to healing our *relationships* with our Earthmates. Yes, this is true in terms of human-to-human relationships as well and I will speak more in depth about how ANFT-style forest therapy heals this too. For now, let's keep our focus on helping people reconnect to Nature in all her forms.

For practicum, each trainee is paired with an experienced mentor who meets with them monthly to go over assignments and questions. Monthly cohort remote meetings also allow the original training group to maintain contact and support from each other, to share experiences, challenges, and successes.

The monthly assignments cover seven core areas of expertise and provide a standard of knowledge and competency that results in the ANFT Certification. I would like to focus on five of them:

- Forest Trail Exploration
- Tea Plant Exploration
- Exploring the Web of Being
- The Way of the Guide
- Building a Deck of Forest Therapy Invitations

I would like to illuminate some of what this practicum experience was like for me and how each area fosters an "I-Thou" relationship over time.

The Land

It probably goes without saying that the most important part of forest therapy is the land and its inhabitants. After all, these are the beings that will be in partnership with you as you ask people to step outside of their perceptual cage and into a different relationship with the more-than-human beings. The most ideal place to bring people is out into the wilderness where they can be free to roam and meander wherever they are drawn. A wooded area with plenty of wildlife and water is ideal. My training was in Northern California which is an area with beautiful woods and plenty of land with rivers and lakes. I arrived back home in Los Angeles and knew I would have to work to find a comparable place to guide people. Most of our trails in Los Angeles are mountain hikes. The paths are usually one or two persons-wide, mainly through cliff sides that prevent wandering off the trail and many of them are strenuous. This is not ideal for nature therapy. As a side note, I want to acknowledge that forest therapy can be adapted for all kinds of natural environments. However, I believe that if the guide strays from the teachings too soon, something is lost. As the practice takes root in the guide, the adaptations can flow from deep knowledge without sacrificing the core principles. It's essential to intimately know the rules you're bending.

During the first month back at home I took great pleasure in exploring the land around me. Los Angeles is one of those cities that will never be fully known no matter how long you live here. The great expanse of the place makes it perpetually discoverable. I think sometimes this is why the city gets a bad rap as superficial. Through tourist eyes, what you see on the surface is easily dismissed as shallow and empty. But through the eyes of a local, the real city is a multiplicity of places, energies, enclaves, and personalities. You have to find her, in all her incarnations, she doesn't just make herself known at first glance. And so, after living in Los Angeles for over 30 years, I went out again with fresh eyes, lover's eyes, to listen to her story told from her trails. To let her tell me where she wanted me to bring people to reconnect with her. To show me her medicine.

After many trail explorations, I found she wanted to be met in Tadpole Creek, at the Sepulveda Wildlife Reserve, in Franklin Canyon, the Los Angeles Arboretum, and in the Angeles National Forest. All different offerings. All different medicines. For now, I will tell you the story of Tadpole Creek...

For my first few public walks I returned to the Angeles Forest. It truly is a wilderness and offers close encounters with bears, deer, bay laurel trees, towering pines, and a year-round waterfall, sourced from an underground spring. But it is quite a drive from the San Fernando Valley where I live and work, and I wanted to find a place to take people on this side of the city. As I searched every trail in my area, I noticed I was getting caught in a concept and fear that a simpler area of land may not speak to people the way the National Forests do. This is an example of not trusting the land to provide what people need. It also serves as an example of my subtle desire to manipulate the experience, to provide an "awesome" experience for people. To try and determine the outcome that the participants had with me so that they would love it and feel what I feel. This is a very common mistake in the beginning of providing Nature Therapy and forgivable. But it almost made me overlook one of the sweetest places in the valley and one truly connected to my heart. Luckily, like Dorothy in the Wizard of Oz, I decided to return to my old familiar trail. I hadn't visited in about three or four years, and when I walked toward the stream, I couldn't contain my happiness. The land had everything the training suggested, plus so many fond memories. It was a kind of a homecoming I didn't expect. A reunion.

Tadpole Creek is the nickname I gave to this quiet little canyon park, tucked off a busy road. From the street it doesn't look like much and since it isn't a strenuous hike, in fact very little incline if any, it rarely attracts the fitness-minded folks who use the local trails as gyms. Again, there's nothing wrong with getting a workout in nature. In fact, it's one of the only ways I tend to do it. But forest therapy has a different aim. It's about connecting, spending time with other beings, paying attention to what may arise. In fact, some of the most healing Nature Immersions can be done in a twenty-foot radius. Forest therapy is about the length of time spent, rather than the distance covered.

Marley and I often went to Tadpole Creek when she was in elementary school. We wondered about wildflowers and faeries, watched butterflies in the tall grass and sat under crow-filled trees for hours. And in the springtime, we would catch one or two pollywogs in a large glass jar, bring them home and watch them grow into tiny young frogs, returning them back to the stream with excitement when their tails had disappeared enough to signal they were ready to move onto land. Thus, the nickname.

I have led more than a hundred walks in this area now, as well as going for my own solo walks. I have experienced her in all seasons, all conditions, and have come to know her plants, animals, and rocks intimately. Of course, she is ever changing. Each walk uncovers something new, something needed. I have watched her burn down and regrow in the most sublime ways. She has taught me about resiliency and rebirth, as well as hidden dangers and human destruction.

This land has taught me to appreciate death, trauma, regrowth, the unique offerings of milkweed, butterflies, cool running streams, frogs, mudbanks, and a wide variety of trees.

Lying beneath one of my favorite oaks, I noticed how she invited me to relax. To get comfortable. Really comfortable. To feel the strength of her at my back. The gentle persuasion to lie down on the earth under her canopy. Feeling the ease of lying at her roots, shoeless feet extending along her bark and stretching up toward her green leaved branches. I have hugged this tree. Unashamed. Kissed her cool leaves. And rested. Together.

Reflection Invitation

Is there some location of land that you favor? Perhaps your garden, or favorite trail, river, beach? Can you imagine that this place also has a connection to you? That the beings in this place know who you are and are happy to see you when you're there?

Tea Plants

Each Forest Immersion ends with a Tea Ceremony. Along with a first aid kit, all guides carry a teapot and cups and either a burner to heat water, or a thermos that holds hot water to steep a trail plant for the end of the walk. It's crucial that the guides are familiar with the edible plants along the trail and know without a doubt that the plants they choose for the tea are safe. Each trail has specific plants (pine, bay laurel, rosemary, mint, fennel, lavender, to name a few) that can be harvested on the walk.

Drinking tea together at the end of the walk is a significant way to give everyone a chance to have intentional closure on their experience. It also provides another way of thanking the land and taking the forest into themselves. As each cup of tea is poured and distributed, the first cup is offered to the land in recognition. This simple act of including the land in the group as a participant can be very powerful in shifting and supporting an "I-Thou" attitude toward the rest of nature. The gesture of giving the land the first cup of tea recognizes that she is a living being here *with* us, not *for* us. It also subtly realigns us from perceiving ourselves in the dominant position that our broken relationship promotes, and allows us to regard the rest of nature with humility and respect. Connecting from this humbled place of equality is a huge part of repairing our thinking and stepping outside of our faulty perceptual cage that keeps us separate from our Earthmates.

Reflection Invitation

Wander out into a wilder area and notice what plants may be there that you feel drawn to. Is there a rosemary or lavender bush? Sage or mint? Wild fennel? If you encounter this kind of plant-being, ask its permission for you to collect some leaves or sprigs. If the answer is yes, steep them for a few minutes in hot water and enjoy taking this being into your body as a gentle tea. Thank the plant for its generosity. Consider if there's something you might give to the plant or the land in return.

Web of Being

The concept of a "web of being" is a beautiful way of describing the interdependence of all living things. I like to imagine that not too long ago, we had much more of a grasp on how interdependent we are with all things. Perhaps when we lived closer to the land, grew our own food, and knew the rest of nature more intimately because of it. Although we still placed ourselves superior to the rest of nature, there was at least more of a sense of interdependence. Forest therapy offers us an opportunity to reflect on this interdependence but goes a step further. ANFT-style nature therapy is the real-time exploration and deepening awareness over time of the ways *all things* give and receive each other simultaneously as one organic entity. The most thought shifting component of contemplating the Web of Being is to include yourself *in* the web rather than placing yourself as an outside observer. Because of our ability to observe ourselves, we can imagine ourselves inside the entire web we see.

So, for example, I can go out into my woods and simply reflect on the relationships between a tree, the stream, and the sun: the tree draws water from the stream, the stream water is purified by the tree, the sun evaporates stream water into the atmosphere, the water in the atmosphere is stored by the trees, the tree uses sunlight in its leaves, and so on. Now, adding myself into the web, I have to consider what I am receiving and what I am giving. The tree gives me oxygen as well as shade from the sun, and takes in carbon dioxide from me. The tree may also receive any pruning I might do of dead branches. The water keeps me cool in the heat. I can also drink the water (especially off the leaves as dew), but what do I give the water? The sunlight gives me warmth, light, vitamin D, but what do I give the sun? I can clean the water of any garbage that might be polluting it. I can give thanks to the Sun. The Sun gives without directly receiving. Or perhaps I might imagine the Sun, aware of us in some way, is satisfied simply with my being. Obviously, this is a very personal journey of exploring and answering or just living the questions.

There is another level of giving and receiving that arises in the intimate place between two beings but requires trusting way beyond the cage we've been taught to accept as "reality." I will say it simply. When I sit with another being, for example a tree, I receive its beauty. And, wait for it, the tree receives my beauty in return. This is the lost bond that we can rediscover. Giving and receiving our essences, our beauty, our love, our joy. This is the primordial element that binds all living things to each other, and when remembered on a cellular level, shifts the way we treat all others — human and more-than-human. That shift is the promise of repairing our relationship with the rest of nature.

You might be wondering how it can be possible to make a shift like this between species, especially now when there is so much polarity between people. We can barely see our interdependence and oneness with each other. Our human bonds are so badly broken many might ask, "Shouldn't we focus on healing human relations first?" I absolutely agree that our human relationships need healing. Badly. But I also believe that our brokenness with each other stems from our severed relationship with the rest of nature. Our conceptual captivity that promotes domination and consumption has also spawned the maladaptive and anti-social ways with which we treat each other. Unless we reclaim our natural way of being with nature, I don't think we will make much progress with each other.

Another point to consider is that for many people, connecting with other-than-human beings is safer. We see and feel an unconditional acceptance from the more-than-human world. Many people have not had unconditional acceptance from other people. Quite the contrary. Bonding with the more-than-human beings can create a foundational experience that may be extended back to humans. Ironically, our repair with the way we see ourselves with the rest of nature may be the swiftest way to repair the way we see ourselves with other groups of people.

And again, the ANFT-style of forest therapy includes a process of Circle Gathering similar to the practice of Council which draws from ancient practices and wisdom traditions throughout many different cultures around the world. Most notably in the United States, Council is practiced by the Iroquois Nation and other First Nations people. ANFT uses a very simple "light touch" gathering between invitations where each person has time to speak about their experience. Using this non-judgmental opportunity to share one's experience, participants are relieved of typical social pressures to agree, or defend, or censor. Most participants on the walks come away feeling very bonded with the group even after only two to three hours together. Artificial biases and assumptions based on age, race, gender, socioeconomics, mobility, occupation, politics, sexual orientation, and other ways we create separation from each other disappear by simply listening to each other share. The Circle flattens any sense of hierarchy. Even the guide themselves takes a position of co-creating the experience. The guide holds the experience and sets the invitations for the group, but also participates in the experience and shares equally with everyone else in the circle. The guide also sets a tone of equanimity, a kind of warmth toward everything that is shared without being caught up in judgements of "right/wrong, good/bad, pleasing/unpleasing." The cultivation of the group's equanimity itself can serve as a deep healing for a lot of harmful human-to-human contact.

Reflection Invitation

Wander out into the rest of nature and find a spot that calls to you. Notice the inter-relationship of three beings. Now include yourself in the circle. What do each of you give to and receive from each other?

Invitations

ANFT-style forest therapy always uses a standard sequence of invitations to reconnect people with the rest of nature. This sequence is one of the most defining aspects of this model and, again, why I believe it is such an important and reliable way to bring true healing to the widest number of people. The design of the standard sequence, in Clifford's words, was developed through years of deep listening to the Forest. He was able to find a way of bringing people to a state usually experienced after a wilderness experience lasting four days and nights alone in the wilderness, with no food or shelter other than a sleeping bag and tarp. The depth of connection people can make in three hours as opposed to four days is quite impressive and user friendly. The first invitations allow people to deepen into their senses, their embodied awareness and to slow down to a pace that allows the normally overlooked aspects of the rest of nature to come into awareness.

The rest of the invitations are chosen by the guide specifically based on what the land may offer or even unique to the day. For example, when I went out to reconnect with Tadpole creek before one of my group walks, I turned a familiar bend in the road and saw that the land had burned down, unbeknownst to me since the last time I was there. I was shocked. I had been used to the trees being the focal point. The burn allowed me to experiment with a new invitation, "Messages from the Ashes." The wealth of wisdom and poignancy the group found spending time with the ashes and blackened tree stumps, tiny bright tufts of green beginning to sprout, was amazing.

Another example of an unexpected invitation was related to the unique Angeles Forest terrain. There are steep inclines along the canyon trail. Feeling my own body as I climbed these parts of the trails prompted me to create an invitation I playfully named "Force of Nature." I ask people to pay attention to how their bodies adjust and change in relationship to the incline or decline of the hill. This invitation focuses on the senses of proprioception and interoception and is such an interesting way to play with gravity.

I've mentioned that a large part of the guide's skill comes from not interfering with or controlling anyone's experience. Creating invitations is where the guide is really put to the test. It's very tempting to add things to the invitation in hopes that people will "get something" from it. But the guiding rule is the simpler the better. Choosing a sense as the focal point, and then inviting the group to wander out and experience that sense in relation to another being, brings the essence of the experience, without any interference from the guide. For example, "Wander out to the lake and find a spot you feel drawn to; spend fifteen minutes seeing the water." The simplicity of the invitation allows an acceptance of the broadest, most unpredictable experiences and really lets each person lean into their own relationship, in this case with the lake. On one of my solo walks, as I sat under a tree next to a small lake gazing at the reflections and occasional ripples, I was startled to see small perfect circles forming in the water. The circles silently appeared and disappeared here and there in a fascinating pattern that began to increase over time. I was so charmed that it took me several minutes to realize it was raining.

The final rule of creating invitations is, have fun. If you're not having fun, something's wrong! This sounds simple, but honestly takes the most time to truly relax into. Again, initially the guide takes on too much responsibility for what is happening between the people and the rest of nature. But as the guide gets comfortable trusting the land, trusting the trail, trusting the actual relationship the more-than-human world is so willing and able to provide humans, the more fun is found.

Reflection Invitation

Wander out into the rest of nature. Find a being that you feel curious about. Is there some form of sensory connection that arises between the two of you? Consider connecting with one of your senses that you wouldn't normally use, for example taste, smell, or touch.

Awarenesses and First Walks

It feels important at this point to talk about the wilderness in her entirety and not just let our relationship with the rest of nature get reduced into a cheap Hollywood romance movie. The wilderness isn't only a peaceful loving playground for us to enjoy. That's the cage talking again. No, the rest of nature can also be dangerous, deadly, challenging, serious and undoubtedly demanding of respect. The closer your relationship gets, the more valuable and beautiful all facets and experiences of nature become. You can be certain that whatever your personal relationship with the rest of nature, needs will be provided. Nature will give you the "medicine" you need to come back into a healthy alignment.

At the beginning of each walk, the guide will orient the group to the land's "awarenesses," which otherwise might be called dangers or hazards. Can you sense the difference in using the word "awareness" rather than "danger"? The word awareness points to the respectful relationship we need to develop with these other beings. A danger or hazard is an objectifying word. Whereas understanding the beings we need to be aware of as we encounter the land develops that I-thou attitude. In California, depending on the trail, we most often need to be aware of poison oak, snakes, bears, coyotes, bobcats, cactus needles, wasps, hornets, bees, black widows, and tics. The guide, being familiar with the area, will tell the group which of these beings live there.

Everyone is responsible for their own body. And if something is encountered, we share that with the rest of the group. For example, pointing out any poison oak that might be hard to see.

All guides have a certification in Wilderness First Aid (WFA) — yes, I can make a splint out of folders, backpacks, and clothing — and know how to respond to emergency situations if needed. We also carry emergency first aid kits. In addition to knowing how to confidently respond to things that may arise, understanding how to relate to other beings on *their* terms, not human terms, is also part of the repair.

There have been several occasions where I've witnessed people engage with another being without the slightest recognition that it wasn't a human, and it wasn't a toy. For example, oftentimes people will want to touch snakes, especially baby snakes, or get close to them to take a picture. Venomous baby snakes like rattlers still bite (but don't have enough rattle to warn). Even though we think they are "cute," they need full respect and a wide berth.

Healthy relating is not Hallmark relating. And definitely not Disney relating.

My first two walks that I led in Los Angeles during my practicum were outstanding in correcting any Pollyanna ideas I may have had about reconnecting to the rest of nature on her terms.

In preparation to lead a group of strangers, I asked my family to let me guide them along the trails in Monrovia Canyon Park. The park is something like a series of canyon trails that ascend through several leveled plateaus where you can spread out and experience the land. As we made our way up to another plateau, we noticed a small group of people pointing and taking pictures. Down in the canyon below us we saw what all the excitement was about. A medium-sized black bear was looking for food among the trees and shrubs. From what seemed to be a safe distance, the onlookers continued to watch the bear the way you might imagine people do at a zoo. However, this was no enclosure. Though the bear was aware of human presence, which is safer than if startled, it also had no intention of altering its terms for any of us and soon picked up speed, moving quickly in our direction to clamber the face of the canyon and up onto the path where we stood. People scattered. And the bear began following the narrow trail up to the next part of the canyon. He steadily approached directly behind my group. There was no way around it. We were about to meet the bear.

With my training, I had been taught that we should make ourselves look bigger than we were, for instance by standing together near a tree. I brought my group to the first large tree I saw standing beside a small cave off the trail and we huddled together not knowing what to expect next. We assumed the bear would stick to the trail away from where we stood and pass by. However, instead of continuing up the trail, the bear turned directly toward us. We froze. And watched the bear sauntering closer until it was about five feet away from where we stood holding our breaths. Seemingly unconcerned with our presence so close, the bear climbed with amazing agility straight up the face of the cliff to our left and up onto the next wooded level where it could continue foraging. We breathed a sigh of relief, laughing in disbelief, and felt the exhilaration of this close encounter. But not one of us denied that this was a lucky one. The bears here, accustomed to humans, are unphased and disinterested. Nonetheless, we knew without a doubt, we were in the bear's home, not the other way around.

The next encounter I had was not so lucky.

The next day I felt comfortable back at Monrovia Canyon Park and was happy to lead a Meetup group that had chosen Forest Bathing as one of their outings. I felt excited and familiar with the land (after all, I had successfully protected yesterday's group from a bear). I knew where I wanted to take them, which invitations I would offer, and had a good sense of how much time each invitation should take to complete the experience in three hours. One of the special features about Monrovia Canyon is the year-round waterfall at the end of the trail. Quite special here in Los Angeles where the other falls are rain dependent and often just trickle, this fall is sourced from an underground spring and therefore splashes perpetually.

For the last invitation I offered the group 20 minutes of "Sit Spot" anywhere around the waterfall. This invitation is simply to find a spot and sit with the more-than-human beings. Some people like to journal at this point. Others just lie down and take the rest of nature in. I went down stream to set up our closing tea ceremony. I found a quiet spot next to the stream, off the trail where I felt we could sit together and have tea without being interrupted by people. I carefully laid out a small cloth, set the teapot out and encircled it with small ceramic cups, one for each of us, and one for the land. It's also part of our tradition to decorate with leaves, rocks, flowers, or other natural elements. They are simple but beautiful centerpieces when finished. As I knelt to add something to the circle of cups, two men came walking brusquely toward me, narrowly avoided my centerpiece and splashed heavily across the stream and over a log in the water. Annoyed and upset by their lack of respect, I turned back to creating the centerpiece. Suddenly, I felt a searing sensation on my back. A few seconds later another, then another. As it dawned on me that I was being attacked by flying creatures, I felt the stings around my ears and neck and slowly accepted the truth that the attack was not a bee and was not going to stop. I stood up and began walking quickly back to where I'd left my people, sitting and basking in the afternoon sun. I covered my head and face with my scarf and as my group started to approach me, I yelled out, "Go back! Hornets!" I threw my outer shirt off and onto the ground and flung my scarf away from me as I crossed into the stream. I splashed myself with water in the hopes it would dissuade the hornets from continuing to attack. I had no idea what I was doing. I think in some way I was trying to blend in with the water. I only guessed at what might signal to them that I was leaving, harmless, nothing for them to feel endangered by. I also knew that unlike bees, each of them could sting multiple times and they would sting me as long as they liked. They would drive me away until they felt satisfied. I crossed to the other side of the stream, terrified they would follow me forever, but thankfully the hornets were no longer targeting me. Instead, they remained intent on killing my scarf. My group stood near me on the safe side of the stream, and we watched as the swarm stung again and again, until my motionless scarf was defeated. Then one by one the hornets flew back to their nest under the log the two men had trampled over. The serenity of the woods returned. Tranquility.

I stood shaking, the stings on my back, stomach, neck, ears, head turning into painful welts, 11 of them. I laughed, "Well, that was something wasn't it?" With care and concern for me the group asked what to do next. I asked if they might gather up the teapot and cups and move with me to a safer spot. I was honestly too afraid to go back near the log where the attack had begun. We found a safer open place and finished our tea ceremony ... a little behind schedule, but what an adventure.

Back home, I unpacked my things, surveyed my welts, and counted them again. The number of stings was bringing on flu-like symptoms. Luckily, I don't have an allergy to the venom. I took Benadryl and called a fellow guide to ask what he knew about hornet sting remedies and another dear friend who has an expertise in homeopathic remedies. The advice was chew tobacco (of which I had none), and Vespa alternating with Apis (which I now carry in my first aid kit). The stings were quite painful and lasted around a week before settling down. I was truly grateful they hadn't attacked anyone else, and knowing I really had only been lucky that they took off after my scarf, I immediately went on a search for what to do if you're attacked by wasps or hornets. In case you're curious, there's nothing you can do. They are highly intelligent and diligent at self-protection when feeling threatened or agitated. They will follow you, find you, wait for you and drive you as far away as they feel like or kill you, whichever comes first. The only advice given is stay calm, and don't swat at them. You want to communicate something like, "Hey, friends, let's all relax." Pretty hard to do. Some suggest running very fast in a straight line while they chase you and then making a sharp turn and hiding. No, really.

Over the years I've wondered what medicine this was for me. That day I looked at it as an initiation into the hornet tribe. Only the females sting. Since I didn't die, I took it as a compliment. About a year later, though, it occurred to me as a teaching in resilience. I remembered their upset, their swift response, and then their return to quiet and calm. Very Zen. I try to let go as easily when something threatens me; respond swiftly and completely and return to quiet. And lately I've been thinking about it in terms of bravery, instinct, and respect. I expect the lessons in that one encounter may continue to unfold over my lifetime.

Reflection Invitation

Is there anything that frightens you about the wilderness? Have you had any experiences where you felt in danger, vulnerable or unwelcome? Were you taught anything negative or frightening about the wild? Notice how this influences or prevents your relationships with the more-than-human beings.

8

Helping Others Step Outside the Cage: Feeling "Crazy, Silly, Stupid, Weird..."

> *I have refused to live locked in the orderly house of reasons and proofs.*
>
> Mary Oliver, American poet

It's not unusual for people to judge themselves. In my therapy practice I work with people almost every day on letting go of the subtle and not so subtle ways they judge and criticize themselves. I believe that humans are the only beings on this planet stuck with a mind that turns on itself. Unfortunately, this self-attack mechanism can also be used by others to shape our beliefs, and our perceptual cage, by judging and shaming each other. Because of that fear of others' ridicule, the resistance to changing beliefs about nature and our place in it may ultimately stem from a resistance to feeling shamed or outcast. Shaming someone for their differences is how the group can control homeostasis. In other words, shaming leads to taming. I am using the word "taming" to mean conforming to culturally approved beliefs. As this relates to the human-nature relationship, our current taming would have us believe we are separate from and superior to the rest of nature. This precept has led to our human compliance with behaviors that have gotten us to the point we find ourselves in now, facing a climate crisis and the threat to our own survival as a species, not to mention the threat to other species of all kinds as well.

We may want to use the word "tame" to distinguish the world we usually operate in from the wilderness. For example, noticing the sounds that come from the tamed world (cars, airplanes, leaf blowers), and the sounds that come from the untamed world (birds, rustling leaves in the wind, water flowing over rocks). As we reconnect with the rest of nature and our untamed self, we can access more than only what exists in our tamed world view.

The good news is, we're able to observe our own thoughts (to perceive our perceptions) and to change them. We can let go of this kind of judging, critical, shaming inner self-talk, especially if, upon reflection, we see it isn't serving us personally or societally. We can change what we think, even if it goes against the group. As more people step courageously and unashamedly into connection with nature, it paves the way for all of us to remember and enjoy our natural way of being in the world. We can give each other permission and encouragement to re-wild ourselves.

That said, when people are given a forest therapy invitation that is outside the normal construct and designed to allow them to connect with nature in a new way, it's appropriate that it might be accompanied by negative thoughts like "I feel crazy, silly, stupid, weird" or other inhibiting thoughts. You may find you have them too. It's totally normal. It's totally okay. This is your first glimpse at where you are in your relationship with the rest of nature. For example, one of the standard invitations is "Meet a Tree" in which you are invited to wander out and find a tree that you want to meet. The instructions include approaching this tree like you would approach a friendly stranger. To introduce yourself and see what arises as you spend twenty minutes together.

On my first walk, when given this invitation, I could feel the level of self-consciousness in me. I wondered, "What am I doing? What's supposed to happen? Am I pretending? Why are there so many ants? I don't want them crawling on me. Am I still talking to the tree? When will this be over? Clearly, I don't know how to do this right." I felt awkward. And although I thought I felt a lot of kinship with nature, the other beings were clearly strange to me. Objects. I didn't know how to relate to them yet. Like talking to a spoon. Why would you do that? That's crazy. But over time, and allowing my inner critic to quiet down, I began to notice what it felt like to be with the trees. Although I haven't been one who hears them say anything (though some people do), I feel a sense of relationship now. I feel the tree invite me to lean against it or take my shoes off and feel its bark with my feet or stroke its leaves and tell it how beautiful it is. To offer love. And the ants, by the way, don't seem to be so irritating anymore either.

Feelings of awkwardness or judgment are fine. What's important is not to let it stop you. In fact, it might be a good sign that you're on the right track since what we're challenging is a set of learned beliefs that have broken our natural relationship with our environment. Our perceptions are the only broken part of our relationship with nature. Our physical bond is not broken; our emotional bond is not broken. Only our way of thinking about ourselves and nature is broken.

Reconnecting with the rest of nature, seeing yourself as nature, and feeling your place in the whole biosphere, your Earthbody, is more akin to remembering than learning. This is a practice of allowing your original nature to come back to you on its own.

Some people have this experience right away and report feelings of coming home or feeling free. Others may take longer to find their personal relationship with the more-than-human world. This is why it's so important to remember the relationship will develop between the human and the other-than-humans. It's up to them to find each other or not. Every experience is right. The guide's role is only to provide the possibility and permission for that connection — nothing more and nothing less.

Being with nature recalls childhood for many people and an original sense of themselves in relationship with animals, plants, trees, water, clouds, sky, insects, air. We have been taught to see ourselves as separate, but in our beginning, we didn't naturally make that distinction. We were naturally curious about our fellow Earthmates and, if given the opportunity, spent a lot of time experiencing and exploring simply for the pleasure of it. It's also important to remember again that not every culture teaches separation. Cultures that live in harmony with the rest of nature and see each being as having spirit, wisdom and an equal place as humans are plentiful.

Most often, healing a broken human-nature relationship takes time, which is why nature therapy is an ongoing practice rather than a technique or tool to use once or twice, or as an afternoon's entertainment. Instead, it's a practice of regularly spending time with the rest of nature, paying attention, becoming curious, cultivating sensory connection, and letting that genuine connection itself re-cultivate what's been tamed out of you. Even our own agenda or what we think we will gain is irrelevant to letting the healing show you what you've been needing. Trust that the relationship itself heals.

As clinicians we understand that what is most important in clinical outcomes is the relationship between therapist and client. Similarly, it's the relationship between the more-than-human beings and the person that will heal. No human interference is needed. It's a lifetime journey, a way of "being with" and "belonging to" the rest of nature that is reciprocally cherished and nurtured as much as any other relationship you have with an important loved one.

Reflection Invitation

Do you notice any resistance to the idea of connecting with an other-than-human being? Does it feel silly to encounter a tree as a sentient being, introducing yourself by name and perhaps sharing something about yourself? Allow any discomfort to be part of your healing.

I thought it might also be helpful to hear from other guides about their experiences since we're all so different. To that end, I asked a few of my community to share their experience in repairing their relationship with other-than-humans.

Stories from the Guides

Prompt: Tell a story of a time when you had an unusual experience with the rest of nature or tell a story about an experience with an other-than-human being that made you feel "silly" or "crazy."

Debra's Story:
Our practicum with ANFT requires a sunup to sundown "medicine walk." From the beginning, I knew that I would choose Topanga State Park — long a site of respite and healing for me. I didn't have a specific place in mind when I arrived in the darkness of predawn. Wearing a headlamp, I planned to let the land or animals lead me to where I should settle. I came to an enchanted looking oak woodland area that I had passed by — but not entered — many times before. This time, I turned off the trail and entered the branched arms of these elder trees. I wandered all the way through and out the other side of the grove, where it opened to gorgeous canyon views and a peek of the ocean between two mountain ridges. There was a perfect little clearing in the midst of shrubs, right on the edge of the cliff and this is where I settled. As the sun was rising, I set out my circle: delineated by crystals and nearby rocks before drumming to the directions and calling in my guides.

Much later, as I was lying on my back watching the clouds move across the sky, I heard what I assumed to be a family (man, woman, children's voices) approaching along a little trail that would eventually lead them right behind me. Obscured by the bushes, I was certain they would not see me until they were right upon me. As their chatting persisted, I thought to start drumming again, even as I stayed in a prone position. My purpose was twofold: I wanted to alert rather than alarm them with my presence nearby; and mostly I hoped the drumming would alienate them from staying in the area. So, still lying there, I started drumming to the sky, singing a soft song. I quickly forgot them with my percussive meditation and some time passed. When I drifted back into place awareness, I no longer heard any voices, but was curious to see if they were anywhere around. Still drumming, I stood and started playing to the directions again. As I turned to where I last heard their voices coming from, I saw the whole family there with their faces turned to the morning sun, eyes closed, and the softest expressions on their faces. The children (around 7 or 8 years old at most) were sitting side-by-side on the edge of the canyon, the mother was standing away from them, palms open to the canyon before her, and the father several yards away cross legged on a bench.

I was simultaneously surprised by their company, ashamed by my original intentions to drive them away, and incredibly moved. I closed my eyes and continued my drumming ritual, eventually turning toward the oak grove where I let my eyes drift open again. The woman had gone over to a tree (one that I had been particularly drawn to as well) and wrapped her arms around it.

As tears poured, I realized I was being gifted one of the most powerful messages of this time in my life: this medicine was not mine. It did not belong to me. It could not be used as a shield. Rather that it was potent medicine that is meant to be shared and the perfect illustration of "the guide opens the door, nature is the therapist."

Some years have passed now, and I continue to remember that day, those moments. And I continue to learn from it. And I'm certain that the memory will be one that I am likely to keep very alive with me for the rest of my days.

<u>Jackie's Story</u>:

I can share three little stories. The first one that came to mind is one I experienced before my training as a Forest Guide. We were on a trail in the Angeles Crest National Park. I think the invitation might have been either "Connect with a Tree" or "Sit Spot," I don't remember which, but I remember I felt called by a tree that was on a little hill, like a slope. And I was walking, and I said to myself, "Really? I have to go up there?" But I went up there anyway. As I was walking up looking at this tree ahead of me, my heart started pounding. You know, not the usual kind of way my heart had been beating. And I was surprised, and I thought, "This is strange." I think I probably even thought, "Am I imagining this, you know, am I crazy?" I stopped, you know, and studied it for a bit, and I thought, "I wonder if it's because I'm climbing uphill a little bit," but it wasn't a steep hill. It didn't seem like a difficult climb. Then I approached the tree. I was just looking up, looking at its branches and leaves and kind of touching the tree. I spent some time there with it like that. And then I felt this pull to go around to the other side of the tree. It was really kind of a big tree. I went to the other side, and I started bawling because I realized that my heart was beating fast and very strong and as soon as I went to the back of the tree, I saw the burns. The back of the tree was like charcoal and burned and I felt sorrow. The grief. It was like a wave that just came and kind of washed over me. That was a gift because I realized that the way that my heart was beating was not random. It changed my initial response of "What's happening? Am I imagining this? Am I crazy?" to "Oh. No. I am called here. For one reason or another, I'm supposed to be witnessing this, to process this grief that is triggered by this tree that's burned but still resilient." On some level, I felt like it allowed me to process my own grief in sharing that moment of sorrow and grief with the tree.

Another experience is one I had in Sugarloaf during my Guide Training. There was an invitation called something like "Listening to the Echoes of the Forest." And so, I took it literally. I got "echoes of the forest," so, I started to hum and make little sounds, to kind of hear the echoes or whatever. So, I was humming, and I was walking along and there were two oak trees ahead of me. I felt called to walk between the two trees. I continued to hum as I walked between them. And as soon as I walked through, I started to feel vibrations, like my humming became a little different. There was a qualitative difference. It almost felt like there were other voices humming with me. It felt like that. Although I couldn't tell where it came from. And I also felt some kind of vibrations for a little bit. Maybe seconds. I don't know how long, but it was so visceral. I felt it. And I paused a little bit ... and then started humming again. But as I hummed this time words came, like lyrics just came to me, instead of just the hum. It brought up a lot of emotions as I was humming because the words that came were *I love you. I love you. Yes, I do. I love you. Forever.*

I felt like the words came from the trees, even though it says "I," it came from the trees. Maybe those two oak trees. There was that moment of doubt of like, "what's happening? Am I right? Am I normal?" Like, "what's going on here?" But that moment was also brief because the lyrics came and then the emotions came and that felt very real. It felt true that, "Yes. This is the message, and it is coming from the trees." And I could feel the love in that. I just felt it at that moment. And my tears this time were a combination of remembering and joy and grief. It was very powerful and felt very true.

Those two stories were from the trees, but the last experience was from the water. It was on my solo walk. I was trying to decide where to go. There was a creek right near our campground. I was aiming for a direction, and I needed to cross the creek to get there. There were boulders and rocks in the water to step on. So, I started to wander along the creek for a little bit. And then I started to hear a lot of voices, like electrical talking or something, and I looked around because everybody was gone by then. For a moment I even thought, "Oh, is that somebody's radio?" I looked around and there was nobody in sight. Also, it wasn't continuous. So, I heard voices, but when I started thinking, "where is it coming from?" I wouldn't hear them anymore. I looked at the river. And I got this message from the water, *"I am the sound of all the voices."* I stood there in the middle of the creek, and that same kind of feeling of recognizing it as the truth in that moment came over me. Now, that time I didn't ask, "Is this crazy?" but I did think it was coming from a radio or somebody must be talking. Once I recognized it was the river speaking, I felt sure it was the water giving me that message.

Ben's Story:
One day, I was sitting amongst grasses on the side of a mountain overlooking the city. I could see the cars on the highways, which from that height looked like ants marching in long lines across the valley. I saw that there were thousands of humans in those vehicles. Where were they going? What was so important that they would travel such great distances every day? As I sat, my gaze softening towards the horizon, I felt as if I heard a voice. It said to me, *"Why are you humans so intent on wasting your time with such trivial things?"* I knew I was alone, and for a moment, I questioned where the voice came from. Was it my mind? Was it my heart? Was it the voice of the mountain or the grass or the universe? Did identifying the voice even matter, or was it the message that was singularly important?

Without any need to reason it out, the voice spoke again, *"Your kind rushes around as if the world revolves around your desires, while the rest of us are teaching our children how to survive no matter what. That's all there really is."* And I felt the grass in my hands, and I could sense that from this mountainside, the grass had knowledge of things that came from their ancestors, wisdom that came from before time had separated us from the world.

What I hope you take away from these stories is the permission to feel uncomfortable, awkward, or initially doubtful about what you receive. Let that be okay. Let that be a sign that you're on the right track rather than a deterrent. In time, you will get that sense of "knowing" what is real. In the same way you know that I am real, even though I'm only communicating to you through these words on a page. You will know that other beings are also really communicating with you. You will remember the trustworthiness of your relationship with the rest of nature. I promise.

Reflection Invitation

What do you notice comes up for you around the idea that you may hear messages from other-than-human beings?

9

Individual Repair: Self-Reflection, Insight and Letting the Land Speak to Me About Me

I asked the leaf whether it was scared because it was autumn, and the other leaves were falling. The leaf told me, No. During the spring and summer, I was very alive. I worked hard and helped nourish the tree, and much of me is in the tree now.

Thich Nhat Hanh, Vietnamese Buddhist monk, poet, author, and peace activist

Two days before this decade ended and we were all about to enter 2020, excitedly casting off the old decade and expectantly opening to the new one, I experienced a series of seemingly small events in my family that resulted in a rift so wide in all directions (myself as the epicenter) that I entered the new decade in a kind of grief/shock, as if every member of my family had all suddenly died and I was left alone in the world. My holiday visit, which had begun enthusiastically a week earlier, ended with me finding myself being cut off for different reasons by my father, his wife, and my daughter. I still feel filled with shame to say that out loud. It was a completely unprecedented experience that I wouldn't have predicted in a million years. It felt as if there had been several landmines waiting to be detonated and I inadvertently tripped the wire to each and every one of them. Once started, there was nothing I could do to stop the explosions, including my own, and any of my efforts to de-escalate things seemed only to increase the force of the blasts.

I arrived back home alone to my Los Angeles apartment shaken, afraid of the level of intensity and the gaping silence. I had been feeling vulnerable before I made the trip out, and as these silent unresolved days went on, with no way of talking things through, I felt a new level of despair. Another wave of loss to deal with somehow. A dear friend encouraged me to take my trauma, my grief, and my questions to the woods: "What had happened? How would I cope? Was there a lesson in this isolation?"

I had done this many times before and knew it was sound advice to let the more-than-human world counsel and comfort me. But I felt hesitant. My woods had recently been through a devastating fire brought on by our annual Santa Ana winds. After the fires were out, I had gone to see what damage might have been done to my trail. I was stunned by the scorched land, missing trees and foliage and general wreckage of broken tree limbs, orange rubber cones and yellow caution tape everywhere I looked. I had felt so much loss there a month ago that a part of me didn't know if I could go there for help now. However, another wiser part recognized who better to have this conversation with than my land who itself had recently been burned down? Perhaps we would console each other.

When I arrived at the trail, I entered close to the road which had been spared from the fire. It was good to see the familiar trees still standing and welcoming. The grass was surprisingly bright green and lush. I felt the contrast of the ache in my heart. I asked out loud, "Tell me about aloneness, tell me about loss." A single squirrel peeked out from around a tree trunk as it climbed upward into the branches. I walked onward toward the creek where I usually begin my visits. A cluster of small trees spoke to me of Family. I felt openness and friendliness as I approached them. I noticed a twinge of uncertainty in myself, being there with such a heavy heart. Was I worthy to be there?

Should I cheer up? I reminded myself to stay with my heart, whatever its condition, rather than my head.

When I lead groups, I offer them the invitation to consider that whatever is in their hearts is welcome in the forest. That even what they may judge as bad, our grief, our fear, our anger, is all welcome. That it's safe to share it with the land, and that our Earth is the great composter... she will take what we feel is shyte and grow something beautiful with it. This was my turn to trust that invitation. To suspend my judgment and open my heart "as is" to the forest.

I heard the gentle sounds of the stream ahead, but suddenly chose a different path than the one I normally take. I followed my heart and was led to a path protected by a group of pine trees to my left. I looked up at the canopy as I made my way through them and saw black pine cones, still on branches, scorched by flames no longer present. Empathy.

I sat down at the edge of the stream. A lone rabbit foraged on the bank across the water. I watched it slowly eating grass. Calm. I heard the first croak of a frog nearby. Strong and loud. Though the sun was up, the sound signaled that evening had arrived. In the distance above me to the right, the familiar sound of a woodpecker. The tapping echoed alone. I listened and smelled the fragrance of the fresh grass. I saw myself alone on the bank yet also surrounded by tall grass. The stream spoke to me about change and constancy. The water moved easily across the rocks. Changing and moving. Yet comfortingly the same stream I had sat with for over twenty years. Reliability. Dependability. I felt my heart ache again and remembered to let it speak to the land. To listen also, heart over mind, to anything that might feel like an answer. As the time passed, more beings came out. A circling bunch of tiny gnats, more squirrels, and birds flying overhead. The grass swayed with the breeze and my nose grew cold. "Tell me about Aloneness. Tell me about Loneliness. Tell me about

Trauma. Tell me about Sorrow and Loss..." I stood up and began walking deeper into the woods where the burn would be.

I slowed my pace as I walked to the part of the trail where it crossed the stream. As I moved, I watched for what was in motion around me. The wind rustled a patch of bright green clover. A crow took off from the top of a tree and moved, black against the sky blue. I was accustomed to walking slowly, but this time the strangeness of the missing trees along the banks slowed me with a reluctance to witness what was gone. Occasional black jagged cinders were the only remains of tall trees I had come to expect. "Their leaves would have been moving," I thought. I approached the stream and lingered at the water not wanting to cross yet. Taking in the changes in the rocks and the lack of grass that would have covered the slope beside the water. Disorienting. I looked down at the dry cracked dirt. Movement. I held still to see what it was. Perhaps a lizard moving through the sticks? The surface of the dirt itself began to move as if being shoveled by an unseen tool. I recognized it as the result of a gopher. It was the second time I had been lucky enough to encounter a gopher coming up from underground. The first time was about a year prior, sitting in silence under a tree, I had heard a scratching sound coming from nowhere. By the third time, I had been able to locate the sound coming from beneath the dirt about a foot from where I sat. Soon the gopher's nose had broken through the dirt mound beside me. I had watched the nostrils sniff the air until a small boy came running in our direction and the gopher dropped below ground again. Now, I stood still, almost holding my breath, and watched as the small rodent burrowed its way just below the surface of the earth, moving and plowing, but never surfacing. Awestruck. As I stood motionless watching the invisible digger, a small group of parents and children came noisily by, crossed the stream and without missing a beat, splashed past me arguing about iPhones and homework and wet shoes. I have no idea if they noticed me, although I stood close enough for them to touch. But I am certain they didn't notice the gopher, gently and steadily moving underground a short distance from where they crossed. "What else is going unnoticed?" I wondered.

I left the gopher still digging and crossed the stream into the burn area. Every tree was gone. The grass, gone. I noticed the same group of kids and their parents climbing the hillside. No trail winding through tall trees, they headed straight up the hill and reached the top easily, laughing and teasing each other. I felt my heart missing the trees, the tall grass and milkweed that oftentimes were covered in butterflies. Instead, tree stumps, ashes, and bare earth. Empty. I walked on imagining how I might accept what I saw now if I had nothing to compare it to. How would I see it then? Barren? Vulnerable? Or would I embrace it as is and find beauty? I allowed the questions to co-exist in my heart. Not needing an answer.

Ahead, I saw two familiar trees that had survived the fire. One of them, an unusual old pine that had fallen many years ago, half of its roots exposed into the air, the other half still in the ground. The tree grew along the ground as if it had decided to lie down instead of standing. The trunk was worn by the many children and adults alike that felt the pull to lie on it. I reached out and ran my hand along the bark, looked up at the green needles, no evidence of any burn. "What happened?" I asked out loud. I imagined this tree witnessing the fire, the flames, the heat, hearing the crackle of the other trees as they went down. Yet she remained. Survived the fire, and her fall. I brushed her needles with my fingers and felt the urge to kiss her bark softly. Then moved on.

I noticed myself scanning the land as I walked. What remained? What was gone? The constant dialectic ran through my mind and heart. The effort to remember what was no longer there became primary, though I wasn't sure my memory was acute enough to know what was gone. I just felt the absences.

I crossed the stream again and rounded the trail that rose behind it. Looking down into what used to be lush and filled with several varieties of plants, small trees, and bushes, now lay open and exposed. Several chunks of graffitied cement and rusted abandoned pipe, formerly hidden, were now obvious and grotesque to see. I felt a sense of sorrow. I stood still, witness to the ruins that spoke of using and controlling. I felt a desire to protect and apologize to the land both for seeing her this way and for judging her as ugly. The thought crossed again, "what if I had never seen anything other than this? How would this appear to me? Ugly? Or?"

I turned toward the trail leading back out to the road. The walk back was normally easy and sweet. The trail hugged the stream and still did. The trees ahead were blackened but standing tall, bright green tufts of needles popping out from black bark. I stopped and admired the contrast. And the burst of new growth. My heart still sharply aching, though not as much, my mind still a bit numb. I simply took in the water slowly moving alongside me as I walked, allowing the questions to be bathed and soothed without needing an answer. I enjoyed the call of the crows overhead. The wisp of wind against my face. The conversation itself had made me feel satisfied in some way. To witness and be witnessed in our mutual vulnerability, our exposure, our secrets revealed, the promise of new growth and change, neither good nor bad. I thanked the land and headed to my car.

The next morning, I woke again with the sharp ache in my heart and waves of panic rushing through my veins as dreamland gave way to waking and the reality of my losses hit full force again. There is a very particular feeling that grief delivers upon waking. So often dreams can soften reality, giving us a break as we sleep, but waking brings the stark truth to mind in a flash that renders one stunned and helpless anew. Again, I decided to take my pain to the land.

This time I chose an area closer to my home. A wildlife preserve that few people know about, where a small lake provides home to several species of birds, mammals, lizards, fish, and plant life. This area had also been affected by the fires, but I didn't know to what extent. The land deepest into the preserve where the water was, had probably been spared, while the outer perimeter where homeless find shelter in the dense brush had been a priority for fire fighters. Smoke and ash had covered the sky for several hours as they worked diligently to put it out.

As I walked alongside the outer edge of the preserve, I saw how the land had been transformed by the flames. Miles of open space now, dark gray ash carpeting the ground and black skeletons of small trees silhouetted among zigzagging paths of lighter ash. It invited exploration and curiosity. A sense of welcoming into areas that had formerly been too dense to cross. I turned off the outer trail and onto the land directly, following my heart and the freedom to roam unhindered that the open space encouraged. I walked slowly and caringly. At my feet, beautiful tender bright green leaves sprouted in clusters up through the black and dark brown soil. Breathtaking. Gleeful.

As I made my way across to the other side, I came to the deeper part of the preserve that had been untouched by the fires. The trees stood familiar, tall; their California yellow and red winter leaves rustling in the wind. Some fallen ones balanced on the tips of the long green grass below their former branches. I picked up a big yellow leaf the size of my hand. "Let go." I matched my fingers and thumb to each blade of the leaf, felt its coolness against my fingertips, and let it fall back down to the ground.

Ahead of me was a small opening in a wooden fence. Behind it, a dirt trail beckoned. I walked down the path flanked by bushes. Above me the sky was cloudy and gray.

Occasionally a bird or airplane flew across the clouds. The birds agile and swift, wings fluid and audible as they beat the airstream to reach a higher treetop or land gracefully in the unseen lake. The planes slow and smaller against the gray, wings rigid, arching toward a far-off destination. I gazed around me as I walked slowly and steadily. A rabbit came into view as I passed the next bunch of dry shrubs. Motionless, like a sentry staring off toward the direction I was headed. Not white, but seemingly deep in purpose, it spoke to me of Alice in Wonderland. Enchantment. Unknown surprises.

I headed to my left, moving in and around bushes in a general direction where I thought the lake could be reached. Suddenly the path was interrupted by a long yellow plastic tape and a handwritten sign TRAIL CLOSED FOR HABITAT REHABILITATION. It sectioned off part of the land right in front of me. I stopped. My heart opened as I felt simultaneously the need the land had for this loving protection, and time and peace to heal itself, as well as the gratitude for having been given what it needed. Respectfully I walked in another direction more difficult to maneuver. I happily wound my way through thickets and tall weeds to come back out to the other side of the path that continued toward the lake.

I saw several inlets along the water. In the first one, five ducks sat at the water's edge. I watched them one by one enter the water and swim toward the small island at the center of the lake. Herons and egrets sat in the island's tree, motionless as the water rippled with the breeze. I moved on to another inlet farther down, made my way to the muddy bank and crouched resting on my heels to sit for a while to watch the movement of the water and the birds. A low tree branch was on my right. Protection. I sat still as a flock of birds took flight together and touched down again in unison on the surface of the water. The ripples behind them widened with time. A rustle on the other side of the branch called my attention. A black-crowned night heron watched the water too. I inched closer and said out loud, "Hello." Turning its head slightly, our eyes met. Neither moved. Simply observed the other. Breathed together. Felt the wind pick up. Heard the airplane overhead and the call of the geese. Then both turned back to watching the water. Silent. But aware of each other's presence.

After some time passed, I felt the urge to continue farther down along the lake. I stood up slowly, said goodbye to the heron and made my way through the grass. Before too long I encountered a lone duck eating its way along the lake ahead of me. I stopped to watch.

Then quietly started following behind, pacing myself with the duck's steady movement. We moved this way together for a while, but the crunch of dried leaves beneath my shoes startled my friend who picked up pace and nervously headed toward the water. I halted.

Then as silently as possible, backed away, hoping the duck would quiet in my absence and resume his nibbling.

Back on the trail I moved more swiftly myself. Watching grass moving on either side of me, green to my right, and yellow to my left. The sound of an airplane directed my gaze upward. I caught sight of an osprey sitting high above me on a man-made perch. As I neared, the osprey caught sight of me. He looked down, unafraid, as I drew nearer. I stopped. Looking at each other I felt his power and confidence. I whispered a meek "Hello" to his piercing gaze understanding how clearly on his turf I was. Humility. I moved on.

Another inlet appeared and I walked down again to the muddy edge of the water. From this angle, I could see more birds resting on the island. An oasis from the rest of the preserve.

Silence. Then from across the lake I heard a voice. An unfamiliar melody drifted over the water from a young man sitting in the inlet across from mine. Unaware of me, he sang peacefully to himself and his surroundings. I listened for a while and then returned to the trail ready to end my time by the water.

As I found myself nearing the entrance, I noticed my heart. Sad. Scared. I hadn't been paying attention to it and now as I felt my time with the land coming to an end, I started scanning for answers, input, wisdom, relief. What had I seen? What did it mean? Was there some kind of sense I could make from it all? I recognized that I was listening from my head rather than my heart and stopped myself. Shifted back into my heart, "Tell me about trauma, grief and loneliness" and waited for something to capture my attention without effort. I walked slowly, letting my gaze wander aimlessly and found myself drawn to a small, bright green bush almost glowing in the late afternoon sun. I sat down next to it. Open, but not expecting anything to happen. Seated next to the bush, I noticed we were about the same size. "Heart over mind," I said to myself, admiring the way the sun highlighted the fresh smooth leaves. The shadows grew long as I shared again my sorrow and need for comfort and explanation about the cause of my pain...

"Stop trying to prove yourself" entered my mind. I was surprised by the sentence. *"Stop trying to win approval"* followed. I became curious about this advice. *"Nothing needs to be proven."* I felt the reliability of the statement.

Here among the shiny, bright green beings and moss-covered ground, it felt true. Nothing needs to be proven. The sun bathed all of us. I let the words settle in. My heart lifted. I thanked the bush and stood up to finally end my time there.

I saw the opening in the fence where a few hours earlier I had entered. I noticed the rabbit still sitting, surveying the land. Could it really be the same one I had seen on the way in?

Unlikely, but then again ... I smiled and nodded in appreciation of him, and he hopped away as I crossed back out through the fence.

Reflection Invitation

Is there something in your heart that's troubling you? Perhaps an unresolved situation or question about you or your circumstances? What comes up when thinking about asking the land around you for insight? If it feels right, allow yourself to do that.

10

The Intersection Between Sensory Connection with Nature and Mindfulness Meditation Practices: I Am the Earth and the Earth Is Me

It breaks my mind to watch my heart and it breaks my heart to watch my mind.
Stephen Levine, American author, and teacher

"Is this meditating in nature?" is a common question. The simple answer is no. Many highly skilled forest therapy guides don't even practice meditation, much less lead their walks as a meditation. But because there are some closely related aspects between meditation, especially mindfulness meditation and ANFT-style forest therapy, I'd like to take a moment to address the similarities and differences. I understand, practice, and teach both, and during my first forest therapy experience had also jumped to the conclusion that it was simply mindfulness in nature. Hopefully, I can help you avoid that misunderstanding.

The most useful distinction is in the intention of the practice. Mindfulness meditation is an attentional skill building practice and forest therapy is a relational skill building practice. To those very different ends, they both develop a way of being in the world that favors sensory awareness, curiosity, empathy, insight, and compassion.

For our purposes, I will touch on a few of the overlaps, but I really encourage any of you who practice mindfulness meditation, especially as part of your therapeutic modality, to continue to discover for yourself where the differences show up in your experience.

Understanding this form of nature therapy necessitates being able to distinguish it from other closely related practices. If this distinction is not made, it's likely that you, as the guide, will fall into another paradigm which may be beneficial as well but would not be forest therapy. For example, meditating in nature. Meditation in nature is wonderful. But it's meditation, not forest therapy. Likewise, therapy in nature is wonderful, but it's therapy, not forest therapy. Refining for yourself the unique practice of forest therapy is well worth the time.

The simplest distinction is remembering that forest therapy is a relational skill. It's about developing relationships with other beings (the forest). If you're meditating in nature, you're not developing a relationship with the other-than-human beings. Imagine meditating while you're having dinner with a friend or family member. They may be observing you as you meditate and you may enjoy having them nearby, but it's not much of a bonding experience for the two of you.

Now let's look at mindfulness meditation (Vipassana) which again is an attentional skill. Mindfulness has become something of a standard practice in Western psychology. It's often referred to as a transdiagnostic intervention. Meaning practicing mindfulness addresses a wide range of diagnoses and their related symptoms. If you understand the basis of mindfulness, this makes sense seeing as much of what Western psychology offers is some form of cognitive behavioral intervention for most, if not all, disorders. In cognitive therapy a clinician would help their client challenge problematic thinking. Adding mindfulness to the treatment plan supports the client in having greater attentional mastery (reducing the likelihood of getting caught up in thoughts), greater ability to detach from problematic thinking (increasing the ability to challenge and change faulty thinking into more adaptive thinking), and, by developing the skill to place their attention purely on sensation, giving their nervous system a much-needed break from thinking altogether.

For those of you who aren't familiar with this type of meditation, I want to emphasize that taking a break from thinking is not making your mind "blank," or "clearing your mind of thoughts" as some people say. That's impossible and not a good idea. A mind without thoughts is brain dead or damaged. If our brain is working, it will be pumping out thoughts. The skill set that mindfulness develops is the ability to choose where one's attention is placed. For example, as you're reading this and paying attention to my words and your thoughts about my words — perhaps agreeing or disagreeing with me — you're likely unaware of the feeling of air moving in and out of your body. That doesn't mean you aren't breathing. It means you're not paying attention to those sensations. Mindfulness is the practice of reversing that. So, as you pay attention to the sensations of air moving in and out of your nostrils, let's say, you won't be paying attention to your thoughts — which gives the illusion of not thinking. Developing and refining the ability to place your attention where you want it to be and maintaining that focus for a decent amount of time, allows your mind to stabilize, function optimally, and have more enjoyment to boot. My personal preference is enjoying the sense of being alive during the time I have, more than optimizing my functionality, but whatever leads the horses to water is fine.

In brief, mindfulness favors sensing over thinking; sensory awareness. Regardless of the sensation one encounters, the meditator develops the skill to explore it non-judgmentally with an attitude of kindhearted curiosity. Thus, the suffering mind quiets down and the experience of being alive becomes deeper and richer moment by moment.

Reflection Invitation

Take a moment right now to notice any sensations that you feel as the air moves into your nasal passages. Now notice the sensations as the air moves out of your nasal passages. They probably feel quite different, which is how you know what to name them (inhale or exhale). Let go of any desire to control your breathing or breath in any particular way. Shallow breathing is just as good as deep breathing. Trust that your body knows what kind of breath it needs. Notice what thinking about breathing is like. Notice what simply sensing breathing is like.

So, what does ANFT-style forest therapy have in common with mindfulness meditation? Like mindfulness, nature and forest therapy favors a sensory connection to the rest of nature and an attitude of exploration and curiosity. As previously discussed, ANFT-style forest therapy always begins by reconnecting to our senses, our personal body, and noticing if we find any pleasure from our senses. The standard sequence begins with Pleasures of Presence — taking the group through experiencing at least five of their senses and acknowledging enjoying them if they do. Orienting people's attention to their senses and allowing them time to experience the pleasure of their body, helps shift them into an embodied awareness, like mindfulness does.

In contrast to mindfulness meditation, in forest therapy, thoughts, ideas, inspirations and other mental activities are also welcome and are very much part of the individual's deepening relationship with the other beings around them. For example, someone may recognize that they really enjoy their sense of smell in a particular area of the woods. If they wanted to, they could "follow" fragrances the entire time and become curious about what they're smelling, perhaps if it's a familiar scent, remembering or reminiscing about other times they experienced it. If it's unfamiliar, perhaps locating the scent and wondering more about its source, or simply enjoying the fragrances as they occur. These kinds of blended connections (sensing/thinking) are how relationships and bonds are formed. The experiences between you and another being are more like conversations, or dialogues that deepen with associations, and a back and forth sharing of observations of each other. Magical things can happen that are quite readily available anytime we decide to connect with the rest of nature in this intimate way. I once led a Full Moon Forest Immersion on Halloween night. Inspired by the holiday, I offered the group an invitation called "Trick for Treat" based on one of the more ancient traditions of singing a song, reciting a poem, telling a joke or some other "trick" to earn a treat. I invited the group to approach an other-than-human being, perform a "trick" and see if the being might have a "treat" for them in return. As we gathered after the invitation, it was clear that the beings truly did have many "treats" to bestow to each person. One of the most remarkable ones being a woman who did a short dance for a tree after which a pine cone dropped into her hand. Truth.

Developing an attitude of wonder and curiosity is another intersection. Mindfulness meditation uses terminology such as "beginner's mind" to capture the attitude one brings to the experience. Oftentimes the practitioner is instructed to sense the breath as if they've never felt it before. The intention is to break the trance of "been there, done that" that clouds our perception and dulls our experience. And breaks the patterns of thinking that have developed to allow for new observations to arise. Again, this skill is particularly useful when the thinking is maladaptive, but helpful regardless for us to have "fresh" experiences as much as possible. ANFT-style forest therapy also encourages a state of wonder and curiosity. Similarly, it breaks stale thinking that might dull the current experience, but it also realigns people with their own innate ability to connect with the rest of nature. The guide seeks to support each person in finding their own questions and their own answers in relationship to the other-than-humans. For example, someone may hear the loud call of a raven overhead, turn to the guide, and ask why it's making that sound. A skilled guide would return the question, "I wonder how you might find out?" validating their curiosity and amplifying their wondering. Following their own curiosity may lead them to go closer to the raven, sit or stand and observe for a while until the answer arises. Or not. In forest therapy answers are less of the goal than the wonder. Many times, the answers only appear after many encounters and ideally would lead to more wonderings. Like any good relationship, we want to keep the freshness and respect alive and not degenerate into thinking we know our family, friends, and lovers so well that we grow "bored," "tired," or resentful of them. These same values of respect and letting go of the attitude that we already know everything is essential to our relationship with the rest of nature. The most certain way to destroy intimacy in a relationship is to project our thoughts onto another being, human or other.

Finally, I want to mention again an aspect of embodied awareness that is another intersection. Awakening to our Earthbody. In other words, recognizing that we *are* Earth. Zen master, Thich Nhat Hanh, writes eloquently and prolifically about Earth as ourselves and the importance of awakening to that truth in order to survive.

We often forget that the planet we are living on has given us all the elements that make up our bodies... The Earth is not just the environment we live in. We are the Earth, and we are always carrying her within us. —Thich Nhat Hanh

Forest therapy also promotes the exploration of feeling ourselves *as* nature not just *in* nature. As we develop our relations with the rest of nature this truth becomes evident. Each practice also underscores the principles of gentleness, kindness, fondness, and caring. These are heart-centered practices; wisdom traditions that teach us how to be with ourselves in gentleness, and with all other beings in that same way. We come to experience ourselves deeply and lovingly, embedded in the entire web of interbeing, not just as a concept or fairytale, but as a felt sense of belonging with and belonging to Earth, our Earthmates, and our Self. Inseparable.

Reflection Invitation

What comes up for you when you contemplate that you yourself *are* Nature? That you yourself *are* the Earth? How do you experience your body as embedded in the rest of nature?

11

Sit Spot: DIY Nature and Forest Therapy

There is a love of wild Nature in everybody, an ancient
motherlove ever showing itself whether recognized or
no, and however covered by cares and duties.

John Muir, Scottish American naturalist

I want to dedicate this chapter to the invitation of "Sit Spot" mainly for the purpose of presenting you with a way to begin your personal journey of reconnecting with your Earthmates and your Earthbody right now. Whether you feel drawn to become certified as an ANFT forest therapy guide or just want to realign yourself and your consciousness with the rest of nature, Sit Spot is the best possible beginning. Over time, you will find your perception shifting on its own and I do believe it will make its way into how you incorporate this reparative paradigm into your life. Once you have a sense and experience of yourself outside "the cage," it's difficult to stay in denial.

Sit Spot is not a meditation. There are no expectations other than to find a place outside that feels comfortable and "right" to you and sit there. This might be in the woods, wilderness, mountain, meadow, stream, ocean, or your own backyard. Grandeur is not necessary. A length of time (20–30 minutes) and stillness is all that's required to begin to notice the many things that make themselves known to you. Our stillness, both inner and outer, can allow other beings to respond by making themselves seen. Animals and insects tend to approach or simply go about their business without fear around you. I will say I did have an amazing experience of seeing a flower stretch its petals in the afternoon sun right before my eyes. I happened to be gazing in its direction and caught the subtle movement.

I could hardly believe it. Or you may catch the exact moment that a branch lets go of a leaf and enjoy its gentle descent to the ground. As mentioned before, the more you attune to your senses, the more you will observe. Sit, watch, listen.

Wandering is also another personal practice you can use right now to shift your mind. Similarly, to Sit Spot, the goal is simply to wander at a leisurely pace, stopping when you feel like it and observing and then moving again as you feel drawn to something else. Watch your pace. The slower and softer we move, the more likely the magic of the rest of nature will appear to us. As we slow, the world can move around us; winds suddenly uplift branches and rustle leaves, dandelion seeds float by glistening in the sun, raindrops fall almost silently onto dirt paths.

You may also like to enlist the guidance of a more-than-human being. For example, your dog or cat, or even a bird or lizard or insect, letting them lead you where they're drawn and allowing yourself to see the world with and through them.

And, of course, children, especially preschool aged children, are natural guides. If you're lucky enough to have a child of this age in your life, let them take you on a journey with the rest of nature. They haven't forgotten yet. And maybe with your wisdom, you won't let them forget at all.

Reflection Invitation

I invite you to notice what comes up for you when you think about spending thirty minutes sitting with one other-than-human being, perhaps a tree. Remember this is not a meditation or a time for you to think or journal. Rather it is time to bond, notice, and spend time with this life form.

12

Integration: The Eagle's View

Life seeks life and loves life. The opening of a catkin of a willow, in the flight of a butterfly, in the chirping of a tree-toad or the sweep of an eagle — my life loves to see how others live, exults in their joy, and so far, is partner in their great concern.

Edward Everett Hale, American author, historian, and minister

It seems to be a sign of our modern times that we need to see scientific proof of things to believe them. I, myself, have a very healthy dose of skepticism, needing more than one form of proof that something is true. For me, it usually begins with an intuition, validated by science, and finally ascertained through my own experience. I encourage that method. Because two of the three components rely on you. Your own discernment, your own exploration, your own educated guess validated by others who have an agenda of verification through objective measures. Of course, we know no human endeavor is entirely without bias, even science. Which is why the final proof lies in your own experience. Your own results. Your own answers.

When it comes to ancient wisdom and wisdom traditions that are re-emerging, it seems science is first in line to experiment, understand and validate. Perhaps this is because we instinctively know how close to the precipice we humans are now. In my story, we, as the planet, "know" what's at stake. We "know" what is essential to our survival. And we are hungry for permission to act on our instincts. Our instincts to let go of destructive processes toward our environment, our more-than-human Earthmates, other humans, and finally ourselves. For we are one and the same.

I encourage you to do more research on how humans are optimized in nature. Optimization means that our bodies and minds operate best and recover fastest when we are in intimate connection with nature. The science about it is growing exponentially around the world. As if we are all at once waking up to our ancient wisdom. Believe me, you won't be able to keep up with it. But do try.

My intuition suggests to me that like the way my body increases its temperature to fight off an infection, we humans also have biological instincts that kick in when we face extinction. Why would we be the only species without it? We "know" what we need and where to heal. We only have to break through our collective story that keeps us separate from our original home and healer. Earth is calling us back to realign, to restore health. We simply have to be brave enough to listen.

We have to be brave enough to reclaim our original nature, to remember who we are. And to be brave enough to trust our own connection in relation with all the more-than-human beings. To trust what we rediscover about ourselves when we are in a loving and respectful dialogue with the rest of nature. To let our instincts, our true instincts, uncaged by the perception that we're alone in the world, fighting for our lives, fighting with each other, guide us back to a harmonious way of being in our world. Trust your true nature. The other story, the one that keeps us separate from and at odds with Earth and each other, is one that has worn thin and is easy to see through and see who benefits from it.

Particularly as mental health professionals, we need to be at the forefront of health. It is crucial that the field of Western psychology acknowledge that this primary core belief must be addressed and changed across the board. We cannot provide help to anyone in good faith if we overlook this fundamental flaw in human thinking, a collective core premise that is false. Humans are Nature. We can no longer maintain our collective denial.

We can no longer act as if a relationship with the rest of nature is optional. This is the next evolutionary step in understanding human thought and behavior. Just as we moved from thinking maladaptive behavior was only in the individual, then began to understand family dynamics and larger social systems as creating maladaptation, we must broaden our understanding to include our relationships with the rest of nature to arrive at genuine mental well-being.

Continuing to fail to include our relationship with Earth in our understanding of mental wellness perpetuates a lie as well as prevents actual health from being attainable. We must, as a professional community, create an ethical and moral standard of care that recognizes and values holistic sustainability, based in a paradigm shift that reinstates us in our natural family, our web of interbeing. This new, old and undeniable truth must be rewoven back into the core of psychological principles of health.

We must also, as mental health professionals, practice what we preach. Again, this is an issue of ethics. In our profession we cannot take the WC Fields approach of "Do as I say, not as I do." Of course, we don't have to be perfect. That would be absurd. However, if we aren't embodying our own best capacity for mental health, what can we possibly offer the people who look to us for help? And how can we expect to help them overcome the inevitable challenges of changing this paradigm if we ourselves haven't overcome our own?

We have entered a period in human history where dismantling practices of supremacy over another is on the forefront. Ideas of superiority and inferiority have come under scrutiny as they should. And we must remember to dismantle all forms of supremacy and domination over another, not just in the human realm. We must also rein in the maladaptive behaviors that allow humans to dominate over other beings, over the land itself. As we are finally willing to call out narcissism in all its forms, may we be brave enough to call ourselves out on our human narcissism, our belief that humans are superior to every other being. Let us call ourselves out on our obstinate obsession with objectifying and using other beings for purposes we aren't even clear on. Let us step down from our self-made pedestal and reEarth our minds and our actions. Like the Copernican truth that the Sun doesn't revolve around the Earth, I believe we must at last recognize that humans are also not the center of the universe. By taking our proportional place in the biosphere we can finally unburden ourselves and have a chance of not just surviving, but thriving and flourishing in partnership with Earth as ourselves.

Afterword: Where Do We Go From Here? What If…?

Once men and women were able to turn themselves into eagles and fly immense distances. They communed with rivers and mountains and received wisdom from them. They felt the turning of the stars inside their own minds.

Susanna Clarke, British author

What if…

There was a point in time when I became fascinated with barefoot running. Personally, I wear shoes as seldom as possible. My feet have always preferred to be free, regardless of terrain. I even became enchanted with the idea that different surfaces of the ground communicated how to walk on them through the "conversation" had between the ground and the feet. For example, a stone covered terrain asks for a slower pace with much attention to foot placement. This differs from sand, depending on temperature, who on cool days allows for speed and on hot days, either doesn't want to be walked on at all, or asks for a slow conscientious burrowing footstep deep into the cool layers below the surface. So, of course when I discovered people returning to the practice of barefoot running, it caught my attention. What struck me most was the reports of people noticing structural changes in their feet the more they ran. Toes began to spread naturally, arches increased, and as certain muscles developed the big toe came into alignment which also helped to reduce bunion deformity. The skin on the soles toughened. It became in a sense a different kind of foot. A natural foot as opposed to a domesticated, shoed foot. It made me wonder.

What other lost capacities might we as humans have? What else lies dormant within us or has atrophied due to a lack of use or domestication? We have been living in captivity for so long we may have forgotten our optimal abilities. I mean this physically but also mentally. When we come back into relationship with the rest of nature might we find other mental capacities that at one time were a matter of course? How might our senses be affected? Our perception? It makes me wonder. These wonderings are for all of us to engage in. What do you wonder? We don't have to force anything to occur. We don't have to plot it out or set goals. We don't have to puff up our chests and make something happen. We can simply rejoin the rest of nature with a curious, kind, respectful attitude and find out who we are, naturally. I hope you will accept this invitation.

About the Author

Julie Brams, MA, LMFT, was born in Chicago, Illinois. She is an Earth-centered psychotherapist, Certified Forest Therapy Guide, meditation practitioner/teacher, and writer in Los Angeles. Her psychotherapy practice integrates traditional therapy, ecopsychology practices, meditation, and the latest advances in the field of neuropsychology. Certified by the Association of Nature and Forest Therapy, she leads nature immersion experiences and workshops, taking people into the woods to reciprocally heal themselves and the rest of nature. She is dedicated to social change and environmental sustainability through re-establishing our intimate connectedness with the rest of nature.

References

Arvay, C. G. (2018). *The Biophilia Effect: A Scientific and Spiritual Exploration of the Healing Bond Between Humans and Nature.* Sounds True.

Arvay, C. G. (2018). *The Healing Code of Nature: Discovering the New Science of Eco-Psychosomatics.* Sounds True.

Crabtree, S., & Dunne, J. (2022). 'Towards a Science of Archaeoecology' in *Trends in Ecology and Evolution* (August 30,2022). DOI: 10.1016/j.tree.2022.07.010.

Davis, J. (2016). Naropa University and School of Lost Borders. https://www.Naropa.edu.

Hanh, T. N. (2013). *Love Letter to the Earth.* Parallax Press.

Hartmann, T. (2004). *The Last Hours of Ancient Sunlight: The Fate of the World and What We Can Do Before It's Too Late.* Three Rivers Press.

James, W. (1950). *The Principles of Psychology.* Dover Publications.

Macy, J., & Brown, M. (2014). *Coming Back to Life.* New Society Publishers.

Roszak, T., Gomes, M., & Kanner, A. (1995). *Ecopsychology: Restoring the Earth, Healing the Mind.* Sierra Club Books.

Selhub, E. M., Logan, A. C. (2012). *Your Brain on Nature: The Science of Nature's Influence on Your Health and Happiness.* HarperCollins.

The United American Indians of New England (2024). https://www.Uaine.org.

Wikipedia (2024). "Roger Dunbar." Wikimedia Foundation.

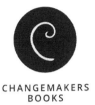

**CHANGEMAKERS
BOOKS**

Transform your life, transform our world. Changemakers
Books publishes books for people who seek to become
positive, powerful agents of change. These books inform,
inspire, and provide practical wisdom and skills to empower
us to write the next chapter of humanity's future.

www.changemakers-books.com